AUTISM MANAGEMENT IN KIDS

Effective Strategies for Support

Peggy S. Ortiz

Table of contents

Introduction to Autism

What is Autism Spectrum Disorder (ASD)?

Chemical imbalance Range Problem (ASD) is a complex neurodevelopmental condition that influences social cooperation, correspondence, conduct, and tangible handling. It is described by a large number of side effects and difficulties, which is the reason it's known as a "range" jumble. ASD regularly becomes obvious in youth, and its seriousness differs from one individual to another. Normal signs remember troubles with social associations, monotonous ways of behaving, and limited interests. Early determination and intercessions can assist people with ASD in leading satisfying lives and fostering their special assets.

Side effects: The side effects of ASD can differ broadly, however, they frequently remember difficulties in understanding and answering expressive gestures, trouble with verbal and nonverbal correspondence, tedious ways of behaving (like hand-fluttering or rehashing words or expressions), and extreme spotlight on unambiguous interests.

Conclusion: Diagnosing ASD regularly includes a far-reaching assessment by medical services experts, including formative pediatricians, clinicians, and language teachers. The cycle might incorporate noticing conduct, evaluating relational abilities, and taking into account clinical history.

Early Signs: A few early indications of ASD might incorporate postponed discourse improvement, indifference to social collaborations (like not visually connecting or answering their name), and an inclination for monotonous exercises.

Causes: The specific reason for ASD isn't known, yet including a blend of hereditary and ecological factors is accepted. Research is progressing to more readily figure out its beginnings.

Treatment: While there is no remedy for ASD, early intervention and treatment can extraordinarily work on the personal satisfaction of people with mental imbalance. Conduct treatment, language instruction, word-related treatment, and instructive help are generally utilized mediations.

Tactile Responsive qualities: Numerous people with ASD have increased or diminished aversions to tangible boosts, like light, sound, contact, or taste. This can impact their way of behaving and inclinations.

Mental imbalance Acknowledgement: There is a developing development pushing for mental imbalance acknowledgment and neurodiversity, stressing the benefit of embracing and obliging the distinctions of people with ASD instead of attempting to "standardize" them.

Grown-ups with ASD: While ASD is frequently connected with youth, it's a long-lasting condition. Numerous grown-ups with ASD keep on confronting difficulties connected with social cooperation and business, however, they can likewise succeed in regions where they have specific qualities and interests.

It's vital to perceive that every person with ASD is special, and their encounters and needs can differ altogether. Backing and understanding from family, companions, and society are pivotal in helping people with mental imbalances to flourish.

Prevalence and Diagnosis

Chemical imbalance is a complex neurodevelopmental problem with a great many side effects and seriousness. Its pervasiveness has been expanding throughout the long term. Starting around my last update in September 2021, the pervasiveness of chemical imbalance range jumble (ASD) in the US was assessed to be associated with 1 of every 54 kids.

Finding chemical imbalances ordinarily includes a thorough evaluation by medical services experts, including pediatricians, clinicians, and formative trained professionals. The interaction might include:

Formative Screening: Routine formative screenings are prescribed at well-kid visits to distinguish indications of mental imbalance.

Symptomatic Assessment: A more careful evaluation is directed if concerns emerge during formative screening. This assessment includes noticing the kid's way of behaving and relational abilities and may incorporate meetings with guardians or parental figures.

State-administered Tests: Clinicians frequently utilize government-sanctioned tests and surveys, for example, the Mental imbalance Analytic Perception Timetable (ADOS) and the Chemical imbalance Symptomatic Meeting Updated (ADI-R), to support findings.

Multidisciplinary Group: Finding is normally made by a group of experts, as chemical imbalances show changes generally.

DSM-5 Measures: Clinicians allude to the Analytic and Factual Manual of Mental Issues (DSM-5) rules, which frame explicit models for diagnosing ASD.

Early Intercession: Early mediation administrations are significant for kids determined to have mental imbalances. These administrations can assist with tending to formative deferrals and further develop results.

Kindly note that examination and demonstrative measures for chemical imbalance might have advanced since my last update in September 2021. Counseling current clinical and mental rules for the most state-of-the-art data on chemical imbalance commonness and diagnosis is significant.

Predominance: Chemical imbalance range jumble (ASD) is a long-lasting condition that influences social cooperation, correspondence, and conduct. It is thought of as a "range" since it incorporates a great many side effects and seriousness levels.

The predominance of mental imbalance has been expanding lately. This could be because of a mix of further developed mindfulness, changes in symptomatic rules, and perhaps ecological variables.

It's essential to take note of that mental imbalance influences individuals of all races, nationalities, and financial foundations. In any case, it will in general be more usually analyzed in young men than in young ladies, with a proportion of roughly 4:1.

Determination:

The most common way of diagnosing chemical imbalance can be intricate and regularly includes numerous means and experts.

Early indications of chemical imbalance might become evident as soon as the initial two years of a kid's life. These signs can incorporate postponed discourse and language improvement, restricted social cooperation, redundant ways of behaving, and trouble with change or advances.

The conclusion is much of the time made given explicit models framed in the DSM-5, a generally involved demonstrative manual in the field of emotional well-being. This manual gives a bunch of conduct and formative rules that should be met for a chemical imbalance conclusion.

As a component of the demonstrative interaction, guardians or parental figures are generally consulted to accumulate data about the youngster's formative history and conduct.

Perception and evaluation instruments, similar to the Chemical imbalance Demonstrative Perception Timetable (ADOS) and the Youth Chemical imbalance Rating Scale (Vehicles), might be utilized to assess a youngster's way of behaving and social cooperation.

The demonstrative group really must consider other expected clarifications for a youngster's side effects and preclude conditions that can copy chemical imbalance.

Early mediation is key in assisting youngsters with mental imbalances to arrive at their maximum capacity. Once analyzed, kids can get fitted treatments and backing to address their remarkable necessities and difficulties. Also, continuous examination keeps on propelling comprehension. We might interpret chemical imbalance and may prompt superior symptomatic techniques and mediations.

Understanding Autism in Kids

Mental imbalance, otherwise called Chemical imbalance Range Problem (ASD), is a formative problem that influences an individual's thought process, imparts, and communicates with others. It regularly becomes obvious in youth, and its seriousness changes broadly among people. Key qualities of mental imbalance might incorporate difficulties with interactive abilities, dull ways of behaving, and correspondence troubles.

Understanding chemical imbalance in kids includes perceiving the signs and looking for proficient assessment and determination assuming that there are concerns. Early mediation and backing are pivotal for youngsters with chemical imbalances. Treatment approaches frequently incorporate language instruction, word-related treatment, conduct treatment, and instructive projects custom-fitted to the youngster's requirements.

It's vital that every kid with a chemical imbalance is extraordinary, and their assets and difficulties can differ altogether. Acknowledgment, compassion, and advancing consideration are fundamental in supporting kids with mental imbalances to flourish and arrive at their maximum capacity. On the off chance that you have explicit inquiries or need more data, kindly go ahead and inquire.

Early Signs: Mental imbalance can appear in different ways, however, a few normal early signs might incorporate restricted eye-to-eye connection, postponed discourse or language abilities, trouble with social communications (like playing with peers), and dull ways of behaving like hand-fluttering or turning objects.

Range Confusion: Chemical imbalance is a range problem, meaning it influences people distinctively and to changing degrees. Some might have gentle side effects, while others might have more serious difficulties. Therefore it's alluded to as a Chemical imbalance Range Issue (ASD).

Determination: A conclusion of chemical imbalance is ordinarily made by a group of experts, including clinicians, pediatricians, and language teachers. Early finding is fundamental for getting to early mediation benefits that can have a huge effect on a youngster's turn of events.

Correspondence Difficulties: Numerous youngsters with mental imbalances might battle with verbal correspondence. Some might be nonverbal, while others might experience issues with language pragmatics, like figuring out mockery or keeping a discussion.

Tedious Ways of Behaving: Monotonous ways of behaving and interests are normal among kids with chemical imbalances. These can go from arranging toys in a particular request to a profound interest in a specific point or item.

Tangible Responsive qualities: Kids with chemical imbalances frequently have tactile awarenesses. They might be easily affected (excessively delicate) or hypersensitive (under-delicate) to tangible improvements like touch, sound, or light. This can affect their day-to-day existence and may require tactile facilities.

Intercessions: Applied Conduct Examination (ABA), language training, and word-related treatment are a portion of the mediations normally used to assist kids with mental imbalance. These intercessions are custom-fitted to address explicit requirements and difficulties.

Consideration and Acknowledgment: Advancing consideration and acknowledgment of youngsters with mental imbalance in schools and the local area is pivotal. Establishing a strong and understanding climate can have a tremendous effect on their social and instructive encounters.

Steady Families: Families assume a focal part in the existence of a youngster with a chemical imbalance. Offering close-to-home help, looking for assets, and interfacing with help gatherings can be gainful for both the youngster and their loved ones.

Exploration and Mindfulness: Chemical imbalance research is progressing, and mindfulness crusades expect to lessen shame and work on understanding. Remaining informed about the most recent improvements in chemical imbalance can be useful for guardians and parental figures.

Chapter 1: Characteristics and Behaviors

Sensory Processing Differences

People with chemical imbalances frequently have tactile handling contrasts. These distinctions can fluctuate broadly from one individual to another yet may remember increased aversion to tactile boosts or hardships for handling tangible data. Normal tactile issues in mental imbalance can include:

Excessive touchiness: A few people with mental imbalances might be overly sensitive to tactile boosts, like lights, sounds, surfaces, or scents. For instance, they might find specific sounds agonizingly clear or certain textures awkward to wear.

Hyposensitivity: Then again, a few people with mental imbalance might have hyposensitivity, meaning they may not respond emphatically to tactile info that normally irritates others. They probably won't see torment as fast or may search out extraordinary tactile encounters.

Tactile Over-burden: In swarmed or overwhelming conditions, people with chemical imbalances might encounter tangible over-burden. This can prompt pressure, nervousness, or complete implosions.

Tactile Looking For A few people participate in tangible-looking ways of behaving to manage their tangible encounters, such as shaking, turning, or stimming (dull developments or sounds).

Trouble with Multisensory Coordination: Chemical imbalance can at times include difficulties in incorporating data from different tangible sources. This can influence their capacity to deal with complex or quickly changing tactile data.

Schedules and Customs: Numerous people with mental imbalances depend on schedules and ceremonies to make consistency and decrease tactile difficulties in their current circumstances.

Visual Awarenesses: A few people with chemical imbalances might be especially sensitive to visual upgrades. This can incorporate aversion to splendid lights, fluorescent lighting, or explicit visual examples.

Hearable Awarenesses: Hearable responsive qualities can go from extreme touchiness to specific sounds (like alarms or alerts) to trouble sifting through foundation commotion, making it trying to zero in on discussion or undertakings.

Material Responsive qualities: Material responsive qualities can include repugnances for explicit surfaces or textures in dressing, uneasiness with actual touch, or an inclination for particular sorts of material info.

Oral Responsive qualities: A few people with mental imbalance might have oral responsive qualities, influencing their food inclinations and resistances. They might be delicate to the taste, surface, or temperature of food varieties.

Vestibular and Proprioceptive Responsive qualities: These tactile frameworks include equilibrium and body mindfulness. Responsive qualities here can influence coordination, acting, and spatial mindfulness.

Tedious Ways of Behaving: Dull ways of behaving, or "stimming," are frequently utilized by people with a mental imbalance to self-manage tangible encounters. These ways of behaving can incorporate hand-fluttering, shaking, or uttering tedious sounds.

Tactile Contrasts Across Life Expectancy: Tangible handling contrasts can change over an individual's life expectancy. A few youngsters with mental imbalance might have more articulated tactile responsive qualities that might diminish as they progress in years, while others might keep on encountering them into adulthood.

Individual Survival Techniques: People with mental imbalance frequently foster one-of-a-kind survival techniques to oversee tactile responsive qualities. These can incorporate wearing outside sound-blocking earphones, involving weighted covers for solace, or participating in unambiguous quieting ceremonies.

Natural Contemplations: Establishing tangible agreeable conditions is fundamental for people with chemical imbalances. This might include changing lighting, diminishing foundation commotion, or giving tactile apparatuses like squirm toys.

It's essential to perceive that tactile handling contrasts are a central element of chemical imbalance, and they can fundamentally influence a singular's day-to-day existence and by and large prosperity. Understanding and regarding these distinctions can assist in establishing more comprehensive and steady conditions for people with mental imbalance.

Early Signs and Identification

Early signs and distinguishing proof of chemical imbalance can fluctuate, however here are a few normal markers to search for in small kids:

Social Difficulties: Trouble with social collaboration, for example, restricted eye-to-eye connection, indifference for other people, or trouble with understanding and utilizing nonverbal signs like looks.

Correspondence Challenges: Postponed discourse or language advancement, dreary language or activities, or trouble starting or supporting discussions.

Dull Ways of behaving: Taking part in tedious movements, similar to hand-fluttering or shaking, and having solid inclinations for schedules or equivalence.

Restricted Interests: Zeroing in strongly on a tight scope of interests or exercises and being impervious to changes in those interests.

Tactile Awarenesses: Blowing up or underreacting to tangible improvements, for example, being delicate to lights, sounds, surfaces, or tastes.

Absence of Imagine Play: Trouble with creative or imagine play, like not participating in pretend games.

It's essential to take note that these signs can fluctuate in seriousness and may not all be available in that frame of mind with chemical imbalance.

Social Difficulties Proceeded: Trouble in shaping companionships or participating in equal social communications. Kids with chemical imbalances might battle to figure out accepted practices and may appear to be confined or unbiased in their peers.

Deferred Achievements: Not accomplishing formative achievements on time, like not pointing at objects of interest by a year or not answering their name by 12-14 months.

Trouble with Sympathy: Trouble getting it or communicating compassion for the feelings and encounters of others.

Uncommon Developments: Taking part in tedious or surprising body developments, similar to finger-flicking or body curving.

Serious Concentration: Exhibiting an extreme spotlight on unambiguous articles or points, frequently to the avoidance of different exercises or interests.

Strange Tactile Interests: Being focused on specific tangible encounters, such as smelling articles or feeling surfaces over and over again.

It's memorable and essential that youngsters create at their speed, and some changeability in conduct is ordinary. Nonetheless, if you notice a few of these signs reliably and they impede a kid's everyday working and social cooperation, counseling medical services proficient or an expert in kid improvement for an exhaustive evaluation is fitting. Early finding and mediation can assist with offering customized help and treatments to work on a kid's turn of events and personal satisfaction.

Recognizing Autism in Young Children

Perceiving chemical imbalance in small kids includes noticing their way of behaving and advancement. Normal signs might incorporate social difficulties, monotonous ways of behaving, postponed discourse, and trouble with change. Early mediation is vital for powerful help. On the off chance that you have concerns, counsel a medical care proficient or formative expert for an exhaustive assessment.

Social Difficulties: Kids with chemical imbalances might experience issues visually connecting, showing interest in others, or participating in imagined play.

Monotonous Ways of Behaving: Search for tedious body developments (e.g., hand-fluttering), emphasis on similarity, or obsession with explicit interests.

Correspondence Challenges: Postponed discourse or language improvement is normal. A few youngsters may not talk by any means or experience difficulty with conversational abilities.

Tangible Awarenesses: Numerous youngsters with mental imbalances are sensitive to tactile information, like lights, sounds, or surfaces. They might respond emphatically to specific tactile upgrades.

Absence of Sympathy: Trouble getting it and communicating compassion for others' feelings or requirements is a trademark quality.

Strange Play: Focus on their play designs; they could take part in dull or surprising play exercises.

Trouble with Advances: Changes in schedules or surprising changes can be trying for youngsters with mental imbalances.

Restricted Social Connections: They could like to play alone or battle to draw in with peers.

Recall that every kid is remarkable, and not this multitude of signs will be available for each situation. It's essential to talk with medical services experts or experts for an exhaustive assessment if you suspect a chemical imbalance in a small kid. Early conclusion and mediation can have a massive effect on their turn of events and personal satisfaction.

Importance of Early Intervention

Early mediation for mental imbalance is urgent because it can essentially work on a youngster's formative results. Here are a few key justifications for why it's significant:

Mind Versatility: Small kids' cerebrums are exceptionally versatile. Early mediation can exploit this versatility to help youngsters master and foster fundamental abilities.

Correspondence and Interactive abilities: Early mediations center around further developing correspondence and social collaboration, tending to center difficulties of mental imbalance.

Social Administration: Early methodologies can assist with overseeing testing ways of behaving, lessening pressure for both the youngster and their parental figures.

Worked on Personal satisfaction: Early mediation can improve a kid's general personal satisfaction by cultivating freedom and lessening the seriousness of side effects.

Family Backing: Early intercessions frequently include families, furnishing them with the information and abilities to help their kid's turn of events.

Long haul Advantages: Exploration demonstrates the way that early mediation can prompt better long-haul results, improving the probability of a youngster arriving at their maximum capacity.

Cost-Productivity: Tending to mental imbalance early may lessen the requirement for additional escalated and expensive mediations sometime down the road.

Early Determination: Early mediation frequently begins with an early conclusion. Distinguishing chemical imbalance range jumble (ASD) at the earliest opportunity takes into consideration ideal help and intercession.

Custom-made Approaches: Early mediation projects can be custom-fitted to a kid's particular requirements, assisting them with creating abilities in regions where they might battle.

Social Consideration: Mediating early advances social incorporation by assisting youngsters with chemical imbalances to better explore social circumstances and structure significant associations with peers.

Scholastic Achievement: Early intercessions can prepare for scholarly accomplishment by addressing difficulties connected with learning and mental turn of events.

Diminishing Optional Issues: Tending to chemical imbalance early can lessen the gamble of auxiliary issues like tension, sadness, and conduct issues that might emerge assuming mediation is postponed.

More prominent Freedom: Early mediations center around working on day-to-day living abilities, expanding a youngster's capacity to turn out to be freer after some time.

Upgraded Future Open doors: By offering early help, kids with mental imbalances are bound to foster the abilities fundamental for future training and business open doors.

Support for Guardians: Early mediation programs frequently offer help and assets to guardians and parental figures, assisting them with better comprehension and adapting to their youngster's condition.

In synopsis, early mediation for chemical imbalance is a complex methodology that offers various advantages to youngsters and their families. It boosts the potential for positive results and a more excellent life for people with chemical imbalances.

Chapter 2: Diagnosis and Assessment

Identifying Signs of Autism

Indications of chemical imbalance can differ, yet normal ones incorporate troubles with social cooperation, dreary ways of behaving, extraordinary spotlight on unambiguous interests, and difficulties with correspondence. Early finding and intercession are vital. On the off chance that you have concerns, counsel a medical services professional or expert for an assessment.

Social Difficulties:

Trouble with visually connecting.

Restricted interest in communicating with others, including peers.

Trouble getting it or utilizing non-verbal correspondence, similar to motions and looks.

Challenges in getting it and answering expressive gestures and standards.

Correspondence Challenges:

Postponed discourse advancement or complete absence of discourse.

Strange discourse designs, for example, talking in a sing-melody voice or rehashing phrases.

Trouble in starting or supporting discussions.

Restricted utilization of signals or non-verbal communication.

Dull Ways of Behaving:

Taking part in monotonous developments, for example, hand-fluttering, shaking, or turning objects.

Emphasis on similarity or schedules, becoming upset when schedules are disturbed.

Extraordinary spotlight on unambiguous interests or themes.

Tangible Responsive qualities:

Over-or under-aversion to tangible upgrades, similar to lights, sounds, surfaces, or scents.

Responding unequivocally or abnormally to tactile encounters, like covering ears in light of clear commotions.

Social and Inner Difficulties:

Trouble getting it and communicating feelings.

Issue with compassion or figuring out others' sentiments.

Challenges in shaping and keeping up with kinships.

Uncommon Play:

Taking part in creative play that is dull or prearranged.

Restricted interest in age-proper toys or games.

It's critical to take note that each person with mental imbalance is exceptional, and not every person will show this multitude of signs. Moreover, a few signs might change after some time with treatment and backing. On the off chance that you suspect somebody might have a chemical imbalance, looking for an expert assessment is fundamental for a legitimate finding and to get to fitting mediations and backing.

Diagnostic Process

The analytic cycle for mental imbalance normally includes a few stages:

Screening: Medical care experts might utilize normalized screening instruments to survey a youngster's way of behaving and improvement. Assuming there are indications of mental imbalance, further assessment is suggested.

Extensive Assessment: A group of subject matter experts, including clinicians, pediatricians, and language instructors, leads an exhaustive evaluation. This frequently incorporates interviews with guardians and perceptions of the kid's way of behaving.

Clinical Assessment: To preclude other potential reasons for side effects, a clinical assessment is led. This might include hereditary testing or cerebrum imaging.

Analytic Measures: The assessment surveys the youngster's way of behaving against the standards framed in demonstrative manuals, like the DSM-5 (Symptomatic and Factual Manual of Mental Issues, fifth Release).

Formative History: Assembling an itemized formative history, including achievements and ways of behaving, is vital for finding.

Input and Conclusion: The group gives criticism to the family and determines the off chance that a chemical imbalance range jumble is available.

Individualized Plan: After determination, an individualized treatment plan is grown, frequently including treatments like Applied Conduct Examination (ABA) or language training.

Follow-Up: Ordinary subsequent evaluations and checking are crucial for tracking progress and changing intercessions depending on the situation.

It's essential to talk with medical services experts for a legitimate assessment and conclusion, as each case is one of a kind, and early intercession is urgent for improved results.

Assessing Developmental Levels

Surveying formative levels in people with chemical imbalances ordinarily includes an exhaustive assessment by experts like clinicians, language teachers, and word-related specialists. A few normal techniques and devices utilized for evaluation include:

Formative Achievement Agendas: These agendas track a kid's advancement in key regions like correspondence, interactive abilities, and coordinated movements.

State-administered Tests: Tests like the Mental imbalance Analytic Perception Timetable (ADOS) and the Chemical imbalance Symptomatic Meeting Modified (ADI-R) are frequently utilized for analysis and evaluating formative levels.

Conduct Perceptions: Experts notice and record the singular's conduct in different settings to survey their social and relational abilities, dreary ways of behaving, and tactile awareness.

Formative Evaluations: Appraisals, for example, the Vineland Versatile Conduct Scales or the Youth Mental Imbalance Rating Scale (Vehicles) can assist with checking versatile working and mental imbalance seriousness.

Discourse and Language Appraisals: Discourse language pathologists evaluate correspondence capacities and may utilize instruments like the Social Correspondence Survey (SCQ).

Word-related Treatment Appraisals: Word-related specialists assess tactile handling, fine and gross coordinated movements, and everyday living abilities.

Mental Appraisals: These may incorporate evaluations of mental capacities, for example, intelligence level tests, to grasp a singular's general mental turn of events.

Parent and Guardian Information: Data from guardians and guardians about the singular's way of behaving and advancement is significant in evaluating chemical imbalance.

Clinical Assessments: Clinical experts might direct tests to preclude any hidden ailments that could be influencing advancement.

Evaluations ought to be custom-fitted to the singular's age, formative stage, and explicit necessities. The outcomes assist with making a profile of the singular's assets and difficulties, illuminating the improvement regarding intercession and backing plans. It's vital to take note that evaluation is a continuous cycle, as formative levels can change over the long run, and early mediation is key in assisting people with chemical imbalances to arrive at their maximum capacity. Continuously talk with a medical care proficient for an intensive assessment and direction.

Chapter 3: Building a Supportive Environment

Creating an Autism-Friendly Home

Making a chemical imbalance accommodating home includes making acclimations to help tangible necessities, routine association, and well-being. Consider:

Tactile agreeable spaces: Utilize delicate lighting, quieting colors, and limit commotion to establish calming conditions.

Tangible devices: Give tactile toys or instruments like weighted covers to assist with self-guideline.

Wellbeing measures: Childproof the home and secure possibly hazardous things.

Visual timetables: Utilize visual timetables to lay out schedules and simplicity advances.

Calm spaces: Make peaceful, agreeable spaces for unwinding and tactile breaks.

Coordinated spaces: Keep things coordinated to decrease pressure and tension.

Correspondence support: Use correspondence help like picture sheets or gadgets depending on the situation.

Tactile eating regimen: Integrate tangible exercises into day-to-day schedules.

Think about tactile responsive qualities: Focus on individual tangible inclinations and awarenesses.

Look for proficient direction: Talk with advisors or experts for customized exhortation.

Tangible amicable furnishings: Pick agreeable furniture with tactile cordial surfaces and materials.

Lessen mess: Limit visual mess to establish a quiet climate.

Well-being locks: Introduce locks on cupboards and ways to forestall admittance to risky regions or things.

Delicate deck: Use floor coverings or covering to lessen commotion and give a gentler surface to comfort.

Tactile cordial kitchen: Consider tangible agreeable utensils and dishes for supper-time solace.

Customized tangible things: Give admittance to tactile devices or things that your cherished one views as consoling.

Obvious signals: Utilize viewable prompts like names and variety coding to make schedules and undertakings more justifiable.

Commotion control: Use clamor-dropping earphones or soundproofing measures for loud regions.

Tangible nurseries: If conceivable, make an open-air tactile nursery for unwinding and tactile investigation.

Adaptability: Be available to make further changes in light of your adored one's developing necessities and inclinations.

Recall that each person with mental imbalance is extraordinary, so fitting your home climate to their particular necessities and preferences is significant. Standard correspondence and perception will assist you with making progressing upgrades. Talking with experts experienced in mental imbalance can likewise give important direction.

Structured Routines and Schedules

Organized schedules and timetables can be exceptionally valuable for people with mental imbalances. They give consistency, diminish tension, and help with ability advancement. Here is a general diagram for making organized schedules and timetables for somebody with a chemical imbalance:

Morning Schedule:

Awaken time

Restroom schedule

Dressing schedule

Breakfast time

Everyday routine:

Begin and end times

Breaks or progress periods

Explicit undertakings or classes

After-School/Work Schedule:

Nibble time

Schoolwork or exercises

Recreation time

Supper Schedule:

Supper time

Feast planning or contribution

Tidy up daily practice

Evening Schedule:

Shower or shower time

Unwinding exercises (e.g., perusing, tactile exercises)

Sleep schedule

End of the week Exercises:

Arranged trips or extraordinary exercises

Spare energy with structure

Visual Backings:

Utilize visual timetables, outlines, or clocks to make the normal more substantial.

Correspondence:

Utilize clear, compact language and visuals to convey plan changes or assumptions.

Adaptability:

Take into consideration adaptability inside the daily practice to oblige surprising occasions.

Discussion:

Consider talking with an advisor or expert for customized direction.

Fitting the everyday practice to the singular's necessities and preferences is significant. Some might profit from additional itemized plans, while others might require more straightforward visuals and fewer exercises in a day. Consistently survey and change the daily practice on a case-by-case basis. Recall that consistency and tolerance are key while carrying out organized schedules for people with chemical imbalances.

Sensory Considerations

Tactile contemplations in mental imbalance are significant because people with mental imbalance frequently experience tangible awarenesses and contrasts. They might have increased or lessened reactions to tangible improvements like lights, sounds, surfaces, or scents. These awarenesses can influence their day-to-day routine, conduct, and prosperity. It's vital to establish tangible amicable conditions and offer help to assist people with mental imbalance oversee tactile difficulties. Techniques might incorporate tactile weight control plans, tangible rooms, and tangible well-disposed facilities in schools or work environments. Every individual with a chemical imbalance might have extraordinary tactile necessities, so individualized approaches are fundamental.

Tangible Over-burden: Numerous people with mental imbalances are inclined to tactile over-burden, where they become overpowered by unreasonable tactile information. This can prompt uneasiness, total implosions, or closures.

Excessive touchiness: Certain individuals with mental imbalances have extreme touchiness, meaning they are excessively delicate to tangible upgrades. For instance, they might track down specific sounds, such as boisterous commotions or fluorescent lighting, unendurable.

Hyposensitivity: Alternately, a few people with mental imbalance might have hyposensitivity, meaning they have decreased aversion to tactile boosts. They probably won't see torment, temperature changes, or other tangible signs as promptly as neurotypical people.

Tactile Looking for A few people participate in tangible looking for ways of behaving, for example, stimming (tedious developments or sounds) to direct their tangible encounters and relieve themselves.

Tangible-Based Intercessions: Word-related treatment frequently incorporates tactile-based mediations to assist people with mental imbalances dealing with their tangible difficulties. These mediations can incorporate exercises like profound tension, swinging, or tangible joining treatment.

Tactile Well disposed of Conditions: Establishing tangible cordial conditions can have a tremendous effect. This might include utilizing delicate lighting, clamor-dropping earphones, or giving squirm instruments to decrease tangible pressure.

Individualized Help: Perceiving that every individual with chemical imbalance is one of a kind, fitting tactile help to their particular requirements and preferences is significant. Viable openness is vital for grasping their tactile encounters.

Understanding and tending to tangible contemplations is fundamental for working on personal satisfaction for people with mental imbalance and assisting them with exploring the world all the more serenely.

Safety Measures

Security measures for people with mental imbalance might include:

Oversight: Give steady management, particularly in possibly risky circumstances.

Tangible responsiveness: Know about tactile awareness and change the climate in a like manner.

Correspondence: Utilize clear and succinct correspondence systems.

Visual backings: Use visual timetables or signs to assist people with figuring out schedules.

Social stories: Make social stories to show fitting ways of behaving in different circumstances.

Crisis plans: Create and rehearse crisis plans, including correspondence procedures.

Tangible devices: Utilize tactile instruments like weighted covers or squirm toys to assist with self-guideline.

Prescription administration: Whenever endorsed, guarantee appropriate medicine to the executives.

Places of refuge: Make safe and quiet spaces for people to withdraw to when required.

Preparing: Give preparation to parental figures, educators, and specialists on call on chemical imbalance-related security.

Recall that security measures ought to be custom-made to every individual's particular necessities and inclinations. Talking with experts experienced in mental imbalance can be useful.

Chapter 4: Communication Strategies

Enhancing Communication Skills

Upgrading relational abilities in mental imbalance frequently includes a customized, diverse methodology. A few systems include:

Language instruction: Proficient language instruction can assist people with chemical imbalances to further develop their verbal relational abilities.

Augmentative and Elective Correspondence (AAC): AAC frameworks like picture sheets or discourse-producing gadgets can help non-verbal people articulate their thoughts.

Interactive abilities Preparing: Showing expressive gestures, turn-taking, and deciphering feelings can further develop association capacities.

Visual Backings: Visual timetables, social stories, and visual guides can upgrade understanding and correspondence.

ABA Treatment: Applied Conduct Investigation (ABA) can be utilized to show relational abilities and lessen issues and ways of behaving.

Tactile Reconciliation: Tending to tangible awareness can make correspondence more agreeable.

Peer Connection: Empowering communication with neurotypical companions can encourage a social turn of events.

Family Contribution: Including relatives in treatment and correspondence systems is urgent for predictable help.

Tolerance and Understanding: Rehearsing persistence and compassion in correspondence communications is essential for building trust and affinity.

Recall that every person with mental imbalance Is novel, so fitting intercessions to their particular requirements is fundamental. Talking with experts experienced in chemical imbalance can give important direction.

Augmentative and Alternative Communication (AAC)

Augmentative and Elective Correspondence (AAC) assumes a pivotal part in supporting people with chemical imbalances who experience issues with verbal correspondence. AAC includes different apparatuses and strategies to assist them with articulating their thoughts:

Discourse Creating Gadgets (SGDs): These electronic gadgets produce discourse because of contributions from the client, including text or image choice. They are gainful for non-verbal people with chemical imbalances.

Picture Trade Frameworks (PECS): PECS uses pictures or images to work with correspondence. People with chemical imbalances can trade these images to pass on their requirements, needs, or contemplations.

Correspondence Sheets: These sheets include pictures, images, or words that people with chemical imbalances can highlight or contact to impart.

Gesture-based communication: A few people with chemical imbalances might profit from learning communication through signing as an AAC technique to impart non-verbally.

Visual Timetables: Visual timetables use pictures or images to assist people with chemical imbalances in comprehending and expecting day-to-day schedules and exercises.

Cutting-edge Applications: There are various AAC applications accessible for tablets and cell phones that offer adaptable correspondence frameworks with images and messages.

Low-Tech Arrangements: Fundamental instruments like correspondence cards or books with pictures and words can likewise be compelling.

Center Jargon versus Periphery Jargon: AAC frameworks frequently Incorporate a center jargon of fundamental words and images that people can use to develop many messages. This center jargon is offset with periphery jargon, which comprises explicit words or images pertinent to a singular's day-to-day existence and interests.

AAC Evaluation: A careful AAC evaluation is fundamental to deciding the most proper specialized strategy for a person with a chemical imbalance. This appraisal thinks about their ongoing correspondence capacities, inclinations, tactile awareness, and coordinated abilities.

AAC Execution: Carrying out AAC includes preparing both the person with mental imbalance and their correspondence accomplices, like relatives, parental figures, and teachers. Everybody in question ought to figure out how to utilize the picked AAC framework to work with significant correspondence.

Supporting Social Correspondence: AAC can assist people with mental imbalance to further develop their social relational abilities. It permits them to participate in discussions, share feelings, and associate with friends and relatives.

Progressing to Discourse: AAC isn't a substitution for discourse yet a way to help and improve correspondence. People with chemical imbalances may ultimately progress to involving discourse as they foster their relational abilities.

Customization: AAC frameworks ought to be exceptionally adjustable to adjust to a person's changing necessities and capacities. This incorporates adding new images or words as they procure new jargon.

Elevated requirements: It's vital to have exclusive standards for people with mental imbalances who use AAC. They are fit for offering complex viewpoints and partaking in significant discussions with proper help.

Examination and Innovation Headways: Advances in innovation keep on further developing AAC choices, making them more available and easy to understand. Staying aware of the furthest down-the-line improvements can help people with chemical imbalances.

AAC is a powerful field with progressing examination and development. It's essential to team up with discourse language pathologists and different experts to guarantee that people with chemical imbalances get the most ideal help for their correspondence needs. AAC can open ways to work on friendly communications, schooling, and generally speaking personal satisfaction for those with chemical imbalances.

Social Communication and Interaction

Social correspondence and association troubles are trademark highlights of mental imbalance range jumble (ASD). These difficulties can shift in seriousness among people with ASD, yet they regularly include the accompanying angles:

Impeded Interactive abilities: Individuals with mental imbalances frequently battle with understanding and utilizing nonverbal correspondence signals, for example, eye-to-eye connection, looks, and non-verbal communication. They may likewise experience issues deciphering these signs in others.

Restricted Sympathy: A few people with chemical imbalances might find it trying to comprehend or connect with the feelings and points of view of others. This can make it challenging for them to shape and keep up with connections.

Trouble with Conversational Abilities: Participating in this way and that discussions can be trying for people with ASD. They might experience difficulty starting discussions, remaining on the subject, or alternating in a discussion.

Exacting Reasoning: A few people with mental imbalance will quite often think and impart in an extremely strict manner, which can prompt false impressions in friendly collaborations where non-literal language or humor is involved.

Redundant Ways of Behaving: Certain dull ways of behaving or interests can overshadow social associations. For instance, an individual with a chemical imbalance could zero in strongly on a particular subject, making it difficult for them to participate in more extensive social discussions.

Tangible Responsive qualities: Tactile awarenesses are normal in people with ASD, and these awarenesses can Influence social cooperation. For example, they might become overpowered by tangible improvements in friendly conditions, prompting evasion.

Trouble with Hypothesis of Brain: The hypothesis of psyche alludes to the capacity to comprehend that others have contemplations, sentiments, and viewpoints that might vary from one's own. Numcrous people with ASD battle with the hypothesis of the brain, which can influence their capacity to anticipate and figure out the activities and goals of others.

It's vital to take note that mental imbalance is a range, and the level of trouble in friendly correspondence and collaboration can fluctuate generally among people. Early mediation and designated treatments, like applied conduct investigation (ABA) and interactive abilities preparation, can assist people with chemical imbalances to further develop their social relational abilities and explore social associations all the more effectively. Moreover, establishing a strong and comprehensive climate can play a pivotal part in assisting people with mental imbalance to flourish socially.

Visual Supports and PECS (Picture Exchange Communication System)

Visual backings and the Image Trade Correspondence Framework (PECS) are significant apparatuses for people with chemical imbalances and other correspondence challenges. Here is an outline:

Visual Backings: Visual backings incorporate visual timetables, social stories, and viewable prompts, and the sky's the limit from there. These devices utilize visual data, like pictures, images, or composed words, to assist people with mental imbalances in comprehending and exploring their current circumstances. They can decrease nervousness, further develop correspondence, and improve perception.

PECS (Picture Trade Correspondence Framework): PECS is an organized correspondence framework intended for people with restricted or no verbal relational abilities. It includes utilizing a progression of picture cards to demand things, exercises, or convey needs. PECS assists people with mental imbalances and deliberately fosters their relational abilities.

Key advantages of involving visual backings and PECS in mental imbalance:

Upgraded Correspondence: Visual backings give an elective method for correspondence for non-verbal or insignificantly verbal people, permitting them to communicate their necessities and needs.

Decreased Uneasiness: Unsurprising visual timetables and social stories can assist people with mental imbalances in comprehending what's in store, lessening nervousness and total implosions.

Organized Learning: Visual backings assist with establishing organized and coordinated conditions, which can be especially useful for people with mental imbalances who flourish with routine and consistency.

Worked on Friendly Cooperation: PECS can work with social connections by empowering people with mental imbalances to start correspondence and draw in with others.

Expanded Freedom: These instruments can advance autonomy by assisting people with chemical imbalances to complete assignments and decide.

It means quite a bit to take note that the viability of visual backings and PECS can fluctuate from one individual to another. A customized approach, custom-made to the singular's requirements and inclinations, is significant. Furthermore, people might change from utilizing visual backings like PECS to further developed types of correspondence as they progress in their capacities. Teaming up with language teachers and chemical imbalance experts can be valuable in executing these systems.

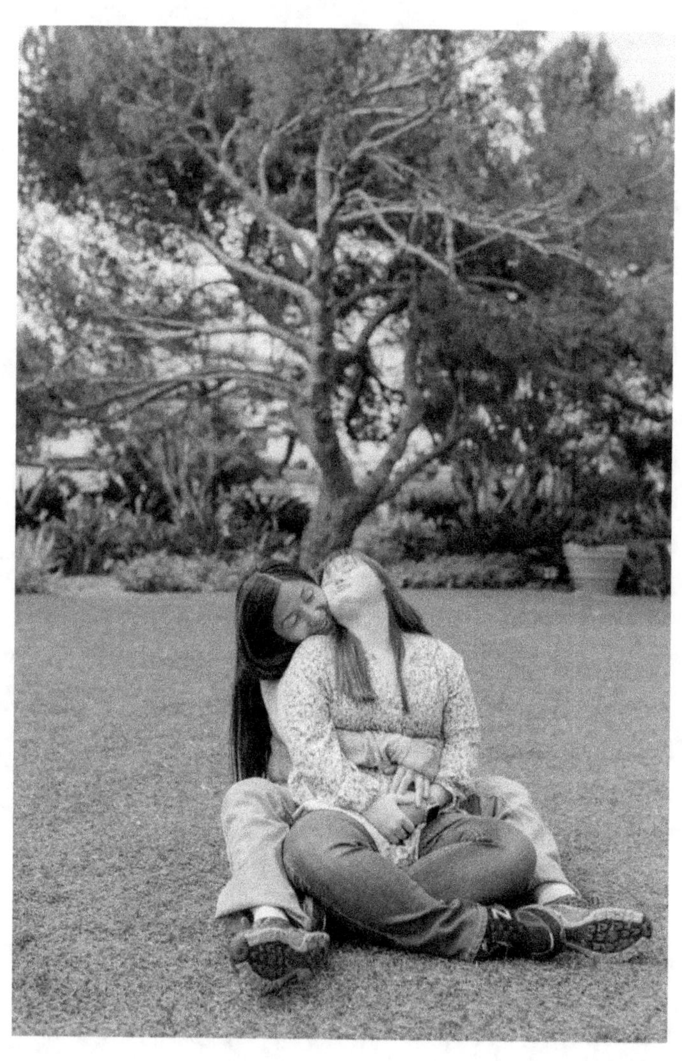

Chapter 5: Behavioral Interventions

Positive Behavior Support

Positive Conduct Backing (PBS) is a generally involved approach in assisting people with chemical imbalance range jumble (ASD) and other formative handicaps. It centers around understanding and tending to test ways of behaving by accentuating positive techniques as opposed to corrective ones. Here are key parts of PBS:

Evaluation: PBS begins with an exhaustive appraisal to recognize the triggers, works, and examples of testing ways of behaving. This decides the hidden causes.

Practical Conduct Evaluation (FBA): An FBA is frequently led to comprehend the reason why a specific way of behaving happens. It looks at predecessors (what occurs before the way of behaving), actual conduct, and outcomes (what occurs after the way of behaving).

Individualized Plans: PBS makes individualized conduct support plans custom-fitted to the individual's special requirements. These plans incorporate proactive techniques to forestall testing ways of behaving and showing elective, more fitting abilities.

Uplifting feedback: PBS depends on encouraging feedback to rouse and empower wanted ways of behaving. This can include prizes, acclaim, and different types of positive input.

Ecological Alterations: Changing the climate to decrease triggers for testing ways of behaving is fundamental. This might remember changes for schedules, tactile facilities, or adjusting actual environmental elements.

Showing New Abilities: PBS means to train people with more versatile abilities to supplant testing ways of behaving. This assists people with conveying their requirements successfully and adjusting to different circumstances.

Cooperative Methodology: Fruitful PBS frequently includes coordinated efforts among guardians, parental figures, educators, specialists, and different experts working with the person with ASD.

Information Assortment: Steady information assortment is pivotal to following headway and making essential changes per the conduct support plan.

PBS is an all-encompassing and proof-based approach that looks to work on the personal satisfaction of people with mental imbalance by advancing positive ways of behaving and decreasing testing. It focuses on sympathy, understanding, and an emphasis on qualities instead of deficiencies.

Managing Challenging Behaviors

Overseeing testing ways of behaving in chemical imbalance includes a customized approach custom-made to the singular's necessities. Systems might incorporate conduct treatment, correspondence support, tactile guidelines, and an organized daily practice. It's pivotal to talk with experts who have practical experience in mental imbalance for direction and backing.

Utilitarian Conduct Appraisal (FBA): Direct an FBA to grasp the triggers and elements of the difficult way of behaving. This aids in creating designated mediations.

Applied Conduct Examination (ABA): ABA treatment can be compelling intending to test ways of behaving by building up certain ways of behaving and showing new abilities.

Visual Backings: Visual timetables, social stories, and obvious signs can assist people with chemical imbalances in figuring out assumptions and changes.

Tactile Guideline: Address tangible responsive qualities by giving tactile breaks, tangible devices (e.g., weighted covers), or tactile well-disposed conditions.

Correspondence Backing: Show elective specialized strategies like gesture-based communication or augmentative and elective correspondence (AAC) gadgets to assist with communicating needs and diminish disappointment.

Organized Everyday Practice: Keep a reliable day-to-day schedule to give consistency and lessen uneasiness.

Encouraging feedback: Use rewards and acclaim to build up wanted ways of behaving and give clear outcomes to testing ways of behaving.

Ecological Alterations: Make changes to the climate to lessen tangible triggers and advance positive ways of behaving.

Parent and Guardian Preparing: Families ought to get preparation and backing to execute procedures at home successfully.

Joint effort with Experts: Work intimately with language instructors, word-related advisors, and social experts to create and carry out a complete arrangement.

Recall that each person with mental imbalance is exceptional, so fitting intercessions to their particular necessities and strengths is fundamental. Talking with experts and keeping up with tolerance and compassion are key parts of fruitful conduct for the executives.

Applied Behavior Analysis (ABA)

Applied Conduct Investigation (ABA) is a restorative methodology generally used to help people with chemical imbalance range jumble (ASD). It centers around understanding and changing ways of behaving to further develop an individual's day-to-day working and personal satisfaction. ABA utilizes different methods, like uplifting feedback, to support wanted ways of behaving and diminish testing ones.

Key parts of ABA in mental imbalance include:

Individualized Treatment: ABA programs are custom-fitted to meet the particular requirements of every person with mental imbalance. Evaluations are led to recognize target ways of behaving and foster customized objectives.

Information Driven Approach: ABA depends on precise information assortment to follow headway and arrive at informed conclusions about mediations. Conduct experts use information to survey the viability of methodologies and change them on a case-by-case basis.

Uplifting feedback: ABA frequently utilizes uplifting feedback, where wanted ways of behaving are compensated to empower their redundancy. This can include the utilization of tokens, acclaim, or unmistakable prizes.

Conduct Decrease: ABA additionally addresses testing ways of behaving by recognizing their triggers and creating techniques to lessen or supplant them with additional proper options.

Expertise Building: A critical piece of ABA treatment includes showing people with mental imbalances new abilities and useful ways of behaving, including correspondence, social communication, and everyday living abilities.

Speculation and Support: ABA Intends to guarantee that recently procured abilities sum up across various conditions and are kept up with over the long run.

Family Contribution: Families assume a significant part in ABA treatment, as they frequently get preparation and backing to carry out techniques at home, which can upgrade the viability of mediations.

Early Mediation: Early ABA intercession, frequently began during preschool years or prior, can be especially gainful in assisting kids with chemical imbalances to foster basic abilities.

It's critical to take note that ABA has been a subject of discussion regarding the chemical imbalance in the local area. A few people and associations advocate for elective methodologies that focus on acknowledgment and convenience, underlining the significance of a singular's neurodiversity. Families and people with chemical imbalances ought to consider their special requirements and inclinations while picking the most fitting mediation approach.

Cognitive Behavioral Therapy (CBT)

Mental Social Treatment (CBT) can be valuable for people with chemical imbalances. It centers around tending to explicit difficulties, for example, dealing with feelings, interactive abilities, and lessening redundant ways of behaving. CBT methods can be adjusted to meet the one-of-a-kind necessities of people in the mental imbalance range. It's generally expected to be utilized close by different treatments and intercessions custom-fitted to the singular's assets and difficulties. Counseling a certified specialist experienced in chemical imbalance is fundamental to creating a viable CBT plan.

Individualized Approach: CBT for chemical imbalance is exceptionally individualized, considering the individual's particular requirements, assets, and difficulties. It means to focus on the region where the individual needs help.

Tending to Nervousness and Tactile Issues: CBT can assist people with mental imbalance by overseeing tension, tangible awareness, and redundant ways of behaving that frequently go with the condition. It helps procedures to adapt to these difficulties.

Interactive abilities: Social shortages are normal in mental imbalance, and CBT can help people create interactive abilities, including understanding and deciphering meaningful gestures, taking part in discussions, and building connections.

Feeling Guideline: CBT helps people perceive and deal with their feelings, which can be particularly gainful for individuals who battle with profound guidelines.

Critical thinking: CBT outfits people with chemical imbalances with critical thinking abilities, empowering them to deal with day-to-day existence challenges all the more.

Diminishing Testing Ways of Behaving: CBT strategies can be utilized to diminish troublesome or testing ways of behaving by distinguishing triggers and showing elective, more fitting reactions.

Parent and Guardian Contribution: Frequently, guardians and guardians are engaged in CBT meetings to learn systems they can carry out at home to help the singular's advancement.

Visual Backings: Visual guides and timetables are oftentimes integrated into CBT for mental imbalance to work with understanding and correspondence.

Encouraging feedback: CBT frequently uses uplifting feedback methods to inspire and compensate for wanted ways of behaving.

Consistency and Redundancy: Reliable practice and reiteration are vital to the progress of CBT mediations in a chemical imbalance. It might require investment to see critical improvement.

It's vital to take note that CBT ought to be regulated by a prepared specialist or clinician who has experience working with people in the mental imbalance range. They can fit the treatment to the individual's one-of-a-kind requirements and offer continuous help. Moreover, CBT might be utilized related to different treatments and medications to give an extensive way to deal with chemical imbalance treatment.

Chapter 6: Educational Approaches

Individualized Education Plans (IEPs)

Individualized Schooling Plans (IEPs) assume an essential part in supporting understudies with chemical imbalances. An IEP is a redone instructive arrangement created for every understudy with exceptional requirements, remembering those for the mental imbalance range. Here are a few vital parts of IEPs for understudies with mental imbalance:

Evaluation and Assessment: The interaction normally starts with a far-reaching evaluation to figure out the understudy's assets, difficulties, and explicit necessities. This appraisal might include input from instructors, guardians, subject matter experts, and the actual understudy.

Redone Objectives: In light of the appraisal, the IEP group sets explicit, quantifiable objectives custom-fitted to the understudy's necessities. For an understudy with a chemical imbalance, these objectives might address relational abilities, social connections, tactile responsive qualities, and scholarly advancement.

Particular Administrations: IEPs frame the administrations and support the understudy will get, which can incorporate language instruction, word-related treatment, social intercessions, and any facilities or adjustments fundamental for the understudy to get to the educational plan.

Parent and Understudy Association: Coordinated effort between guardians or gatekeepers, understudies (when suitable), educators, and experts is fundamental in creating and modifying the IEP. Their feedback guarantees that the arrangement is genuinely individualized.

Progress Observing: Customary appraisals and progress reports are directed to follow the understudy's turn of events and change the IEP depending on the situation. This continuous checking guarantees that the arrangement stays powerful.

Change Arranging: As the understudy advances through school, the IEP might incorporate progress objectives to set them up for post-school life, whether that includes advanced education, professional preparation, or business.

Lawful Securities: Understudies with handicaps, including mental imbalance, are safeguarded under the People with Handicaps Schooling Act (Thought) in the US. This regulation guarantees that understudies get free and proper state-funded training, including the turn of events and execution of an IEP.

It's critical to take note that IEPs are profoundly individualized and can shift starting with one understudy and then onto the next. They act as a guide to offer the fundamental help and facilities to assist understudies with chemical imbalances to arrive at their maximum capacity in an instructive setting.

Inclusive Education

Comprehensive schooling in chemical imbalance alludes to the act of incorporating understudies with mental imbalance range jumble (ASD) in standard instructive settings close to their neurotypical peers. This approach expects to establish a comprehensive and steady climate where all understudies, no matter what their capacities or handicaps, can learn and flourish together. Here are a few central issues connected with comprehensive schooling in mental imbalance:

Individualized Instruction Plans (IEPs): Understudies with mental imbalance frequently have special advancing necessities. IEPs are altered plans that frame explicit objectives, facilities, and backing administrations customized to every understudy's necessities.

Instructor Preparing: Teachers in comprehensive homerooms might get specific preparation to more readily comprehend and uphold understudies with mental imbalance. This preparation can assist them with making a more comprehensive and obliging learning climate.

Peer Communication: Comprehensive training advances social connection between understudies with a chemical imbalance and their neurotypical peers. This communication can upgrade interactive abilities and encourage understanding and sympathy among all understudies.

Tangible Agreeable Climate: Numerous people with mental imbalances have tactile responsive qualities. Comprehensive homerooms might be intended to oblige these responsive qualities, giving a more open-to-learning climate.

Support Administrations: Contingent upon the understudy's necessities, support administrations like language training, word-related treatment, or conduct treatment might be coordinated into the comprehensive schooling model.

Positive Conduct Backing: Systems for overseeing testing ways of behaving and advancing positive ways of behaving are fundamental in comprehensive homerooms. This incorporates utilizing encouraging feedback and correspondence strategies.

Parent and Local Area Association: Cooperation between guardians, instructors, and the local area is urgent for the progress of comprehensive schooling programs. Open correspondence and a group approach can prompt improved results for understudies with chemical imbalances.

Legitimate Structure: Numerous nations have regulations and guidelines set up to guarantee that understudies with handicaps, including chemical imbalances, reserve the privilege to get comprehensive schooling. These regulations intend to safeguard the freedoms and chances of everything being equal.

Peer Displaying: In comprehensive homerooms, neurotypical companions can act as good examples for understudies with mental imbalances, assisting them with learning fitting social ways of behaving and scholastic abilities through perception and communication.

Correspondence Backing: For non-verbal or negligibly verbal understudies with a mental imbalance, augmentative and elective correspondence (AAC) frameworks might be acquainted with work with correspondence and language improvement.

Adaptable Educational program: Comprehensive schooling frequently includes adjusting the educational plan to oblige assorted learning styles and capacities. Instructors might utilize visual guides, involved exercises, and separate guidance to address individual issues.

Change Arranging: As understudies with mental imbalances progress through their schooling, progress arranging becomes essential. This incorporates getting ready for changes between grade levels and at last into adulthood, zeroing in on fundamental abilities and professional preparation.

Hostile to Tormenting Projects: Comprehensive schools ought to have against tormenting programs set up to shield understudies with mental imbalance from harassment and badgering and to advance a protected and strong climate.

Proficient Turn of Events: Ceaseless expert advancement for educators and staff is fundamental to remaining refreshed on prescribed procedures in comprehensive training and chemical imbalance support.

Parental Promotion: Guardians of kids with chemical imbalances frequently assume a huge part in supporting their youngsters' necessities inside the comprehensive school system, guaranteeing that proper administrations and facilities are given.

Cooperation with Subject matter experts: Joint effort with language teachers, word-related advisors, and social experts can improve the help furnished to understudies with mental imbalance in comprehensive homerooms.

Information Following and Appraisal: Normal evaluation and information following assist with checking the advancement of understudies with chemical imbalance and change methodologies and intercessions.

Comprehensive Extracurricular Exercises: Schools can expand consideration past the study hall by advancing support in extracurricular exercises, clubs, and sports, cultivating fellowships and interactive abilities advancement.

Positive Companion Connections: Empowering neurotypical understudies to get to know and support their friends with mental imbalances can add to a more comprehensive and tolerant school culture.

Individualized Progress Plans (ITPs): As understudies with chemical imbalances get ready to change to post-optional schooling or work, individualized change plans can assist with defining objectives and give direction to a fruitful change.

Comprehensive schooling in mental imbalance is a multi-layered approach that requires coordinated effort, understanding, and continuous responsibility from teachers, guardians, and the local area. Its point is to enable people with chemical imbalances to arrive at their maximum capacity and lead satisfying lives.

Specialized Educational Programs

There are different particular instructive projects and approaches for people with mental imbalance range jumble (ASD). These projects expect to offer fitted help and instruction to meet the special necessities of every person with mental imbalance. A few striking methodologies include:

Applied Conduct Examination (ABA): ABA is a broadly utilized, proof-put-together treatment that concentrates on changes in behavior patterns and expertise improvement. It's not unexpected to utilize that frame of mind to show correspondence, social, and versatile abilities.

TEACCH (Treatment and Schooling of Mentally Unbalanced and Related Correspondence Disabled Kids): TEACCH utilizes organized training strategies and visual backings to assist people with chemical imbalances in learning and arranging data.

Social Correspondence, Close to Home Guideline, and Value-based Help (SCERTS): This program centers around upgrading social correspondence and profound guideline abilities, frequently through a cooperative methodology including guardians, teachers, and specialists.

Picture Trade Correspondence Framework (PECS): PECS is a correspondence framework that utilizations picture cards to assist non-verbal or insignificantly verbal people with chemical imbalances in expressing their requirements and wants.

DIR/Floortime: The Formative, Individual Contrasts, Relationship-based (DIR) model, otherwise called Floortime, underscores drawing in with a youngster's advantages and assets to advance turn of events and correspondence.

Organized Instructing: This approach utilizes visual timetables, schedules, and clear associations to assist people with mental imbalances in exploring their current circumstances and everyday exercises.

Incorporation Projects: A few schools advance comprehensive instruction, where understudies with chemical imbalances are coordinated into ordinary homerooms close to their neurotypical peers with extra help on a case-by-case basis.

Correspondence and Interactive Abilities Gatherings: These gatherings furnish valuable open doors for people with chemical imbalances to rehearse and foster their correspondence and social communication abilities in a steady setting.

Particular Schools: There are schools explicitly intended for understudies with chemical imbalances, offering an exceptionally specific educational plan and a low-excitement climate.

It's fundamental to pick an instructive program that lines up with the singular's special assets and necessities, as mental imbalance is a range, and every individual has their arrangement of difficulties and capacities. Teaming up with instructors, advisors, and experts is in many cases key to fostering a powerful instructive arrangement for people with chemical imbalances.

Homeschooling Options

Self-teaching can be a feasible choice for youngsters with mental imbalances. Here are a few contemplations:

Individualized Instruction Plan (IEP): Foster a customized plan custom-made to your kid's necessities, objectives, and qualities.

Educational program Decisions: Select an educational program that lines up with your youngster's learning style and capacities, which might incorporate visual guides or tactile well-disposed materials.

Specific Treatments: Proceed with any vital treatments (discourse, word-related, and so forth) close by self-teaching.

Routine and Construction: Lay out a steady day-to-day timetable to give strength and consistency.

Encouraging group of people: Look for direction from neighborhood mental imbalance support gatherings, online networks, or experts for assets and guidance.

Adaptability: Adjust showing strategies on a case-by-case basis, permitting breaks and tangible facilities.

Social Communication: Incorporate open doors for socialization through playdates, bunch exercises, or local area programs.

Survey Progress: Consistently assess your kid's advancement and change the self-teaching approach likewise.

Visual Backings: Execute visual timetables, and diagrams, and help to upgrade correspondence and understanding.

Tactile Cordial Climate: Make a quiet and tangible disposed learning space to limit tangible over-burden.

Break Undertakings into More Modest Advances: Separation illustrations into reasonable advances, offering acclaim and prizes for finishing every one.

Use Innovation: Influence instructive applications, programming, and online assets intended for kids with chemical imbalances.

Conduct The board: Foster techniques to address testing ways of behaving and build up sure ways of behaving.

Standard Breaks: Take into account successive breaks to forestall overpower and advance self-guideline.

Team up with Experts: Keep working with advisors and experts to address explicit requirements.

Record Progress: Keep point-by-point records of your youngster's accomplishments and difficulties for future reference.

Legitimate Necessities: Find out more about self-teaching regulations and prerequisites in your space.

Taking care of oneself: Make sure to deal with yourself, as self-teaching can interest you. Look for help from loved ones when required.

Continuously focus on your kid's prosperity and instructive requirements while settling on conclusions about self-teaching. It's fundamental to adjust your way to deal with best meet their one-of-a-kind necessities.

Chapter 7:Therapies and Interventions

Speech Therapy

Language instruction can be useful for people with chemical imbalances. It expects to further develop relational abilities, including discourse and language advancement, social correspondence, and non-verbal correspondence. Language instructors utilize different methods custom-fitted to the singular's requirements to assist them with imparting all the more. Early mediation frequently yields the best outcomes in further developing relational abilities for people with chemical imbalances.

Evaluation: A language teacher will survey the singular's correspondence capacities, including discourse, language, and social correspondence. This appraisal decides the particular regions that need improvement.

Individualized Plans: Treatment plans are tweaked in light of the singular's assets and shortcomings. The advisor might zero in on further developing discourse enunciation, extending jargon, showing non-verbal relational abilities, or improving social collaboration.

Augmentative and Elective Correspondence (AAC): For people with restricted verbal correspondence, AAC apparatuses like correspondence sheets, picture trade frameworks, or discourse-creating gadgets might be acquainted with work with correspondence.

Interactive abilities Preparing: Language instructors frequently work on further developing social relational abilities, like comprehension and utilizing looks, non-verbal communication, and keeping in touch during discussions.

Parent and Guardian Association: Relatives are normally engaged in treatment meetings to figure out how to help and build up the abilities being instructed at home.

Visual Backings: Visual guides, similar to plans, social stories, and viewable prompts, are many times used to help people with chemical imbalances in understanding and adhering to verbal guidelines.

Tangible Contemplations: Numerous people with mental imbalances have tactile awareness that can influence correspondence. Advisors might resolve tactile issues to make correspondence more agreeable.

Support and Practice: Steady practice and support of acquired abilities are critical for progress. Language training frequently includes activities and exercises to assist people with applying what they've realized, in actuality, circumstances.

Early Mediation: Beginning language training as soon as conceivable can yield the best results. Early mediation can assist with limiting correspondence troubles and work on friendly communication in kids with mental imbalances.

Recall that the particular objectives and procedures in language training will change from one individual to another, contingent upon their novel necessities and capacities. It's fundamental to work intimately with a certified language teacher who can give custom-fitted direction and backing.

Occupational Therapy

Word-related treatment assumes a significant part in supporting people with mental imbalance range jumble (ASD). It centers around assisting them with creating fundamental abilities and working on their freedom. Word-related specialists frequently work on:

Tactile Reconciliation: Tending to tangible awarenesses and troubles, which are normal in chemical imbalance, to assist individuals with better handling tangible data.

Everyday Living Abilities: Helping with exercises of day-to-day living, like dressing, preparing, and supper time schedules.

Fine and Gross Coordinated abilities: Upgrading engine coordination and control through activities and exercises.

Interactive abilities: Helping social associations and relational abilities to further develop connections and support in day-to-day existence.

Tactile Instruments: Giving tangible apparatuses and techniques to oversee tangible difficulties and advance self-guideline.

Natural Adjustments: Prescribing changes to home or school conditions to help tactile necessities and useful abilities.

Conduct The board: Utilizing systems to address testing ways of behaving and advance positive other options.

Tangible Joining: Word-related specialists frequently utilize tactile coordination treatment to assist people with mental imbalance to process tangible data all the more. This might include exercises intended to open them to various tactile upgrades in a controlled and restorative manner.

Play-Based Treatment: For youngsters with mental imbalances, play-based word-related treatment can be exceptionally compelling. Advisors use play exercises to deal with different abilities, including social cooperation, correspondence, and fine-coordinated movements.

Correspondence Backing: Word-related specialists can help people with chemical imbalances in creating relational abilities. They might utilize methods like picture correspondence frameworks or augmentative and elective correspondence (AAC) gadgets.

Change Arranging: Word-related advisors can assist more seasoned people with chemical imbalances progress to adulthood by chipping away at abilities fundamental for autonomous living, work, and advanced education.

Self-Guideline: Numerous people with mental imbalances battle with self-guideline. Word-related advisors assist them with learning systems to deal with feelings and tangible reactions, which can further develop conduct and personal satisfaction.

Parent and Guardian Training: Word-related specialists frequently work intimately with guardians and guardians, giving direction and systems to help the singular's advancement at home and in day-to-day schedules.

School-Based Administrations: Word-related specialists might team up with teachers to establish comprehensive homeroom conditions that oblige the tactile and formative requirements of understudies with a chemical imbalance.

It's critical to take note that the particular intercessions and objectives of word-related treatment will differ contingent upon the singular's age, capacities, and extraordinary difficulties. An exhaustive evaluation is commonly directed to decide the most fitting treatment plan.

Physical Therapy

Active recuperation can be helpful for people with mental imbalance range jumble (ASD) to address explicit engine and tactile difficulties they might confront. It can assist with further developing coordination, balance, muscle strength, and tactile joining. Nonetheless, the viability of active recuperation might shift from one individual to another, as the necessities of people with ASD can be different. It's fundamental for specialists to fit their ways to deal with the novel capacities and responsive qualities of every person. Cooperative, multidisciplinary care including discourse and word-related specialists may likewise be important to offer exhaustive help for people with ASD.

Individualized Approach: Actual specialists frequently make altered treatment plans given the particular requirements and capacities of the individual with a chemical imbalance. This could include tending to net coordinated movements, fine coordinated movements, stance, and portability challenges.

Tangible Joining: Numerous people with mental imbalances have tactile awareness. Actual advisors can deal with tangible incorporation strategies to assist individuals with better handling tactile data, which can work on their general coordinated abilities and coordination.

Correspondence: Correspondence and social collaboration can be worked on through active recuperation. A few exercises might zero in on non-verbal correspondence, non-verbal communication, and interactive abilities, assisting people with ASD to connect all the more with others.

Exercise and Wellness: Advancing active work and wellness is a significant part of non-intrusive treatment. Ordinary activity can emphatically affect mindset, conduct, and in general prosperity for people with chemical imbalances.

Parent/Guardian Contribution: Advisors frequently include guardians and parental figures in the treatment cycle, showing them activities and techniques that can be gone on at home to build up progress.

Conduct Contemplations: Actual advisors should know about social difficulties normal in mental imbalance, for example, tactile implosions or protection from change. They can adjust their ways of dealing with these difficulties.

Joint effort: Viable consideration for people with chemical imbalances frequently includes cooperation with different experts, including language teachers, word-related specialists, and conduct advisors, to give an all-encompassing way to deal with treatment.

Assistive Gadgets: now and again, actual specialists might suggest the utilization of assistive gadgets like supports, orthotics, or versatility helps to improve portability and autonomy.

Recall that the particular objectives and procedures of non-intrusive treatment will rely upon the singular's one-of-a-kind necessities and qualities. Consequently, it's significant for specialists to survey every individual with chemical imbalance exhaustively and make a customized plan to address their particular difficulties and objectives.

Play-Based Interventions

Play-based mediations are in many cases utilized in the treatment of chemical imbalance range jumble (ASD) to advance social, correspondence, and conduct abilities in youngsters with mental imbalance. These mediations tackle the regular tendency of youngsters to participate in play exercises and use them as helpful devices. Here are a few central issues about play-based mediation in chemical imbalance:

Interactive ability Advancement: Play-based mediations expect to work on friendly communications and companion connections. Through directed play, youngsters with mental imbalances figure out how to alternate, share, and participate in proportional play, which can be trying for them.

Relational abilities: Play gives a setting to correspondence. Discourse and language specialists frequently integrate play into their meetings to empower verbal correspondence or elective specialized techniques like signals or visual guides.

Creative Mind and Innovativeness: Play-based mediation can assist kids with mental imbalance and foster their creative minds and imagination. Exercises like imagine play or inventive narrating can be integrated to invigorate these abilities.

Diminishing Generalized Ways of Behaving: Taking part in organized play exercises can assist with decreasing dull or generalized ways of behaving regularly found in chemical imbalance, as it gives an elective focal point of consideration.

Parent Association: Many play-based mediations include guardians or guardians. This permits them to figure out how to draw in with their kid in significant play and persist the abilities acquired in treatment into the home climate.

Applied Conduct Examination (ABA): ABA treatment frequently incorporates play-based methods to show new abilities and support wanted ways of behaving in youngsters with mental imbalance.

Individualized Approach: Play-based intercessions are normally custom-made to the particular requirements and interests of the kid. What works for one kid with a chemical imbalance may not be successful for another, so individualization is pivotal.

Organized Play: While play is innately fun, organized play is intended to have explicit restorative objectives. Advisors cautiously plan and guide the play exercises to accomplish these objectives.

Early Mediation: Beginning play-based intercessions early, preferably during the preschool years, can be especially gainful as it can assist with tending to formative deferrals and work on long-haul results.

Proof Based: Many play-based mediations have been contemplated and viewed as compelling in working on friendly and relational abilities in youngsters with mental imbalances. Nonetheless, the decision of intercession ought to be founded on the singular youngster's requirements and assets.

It's essential to take note that while play-based mediations can be exceptionally viable, they are much of the time only one part of an exhaustive treatment plan for a chemical imbalance, which may likewise incorporate different treatments, instructive help, and family contribution. Guardians and parental figures ought to work intimately with experts to decide the most fitting mediation for their youngster's one-of-a-kind requirements.

Music Therapy

Music treatment can be valuable for people with mental imbalances. It can assist with further developing relational abilities, decrease uneasiness, and upgrade social collaborations. Music specialists utilize different strategies like mood, tone, and ad-lib to address explicit objectives customized to the singular's requirements. Research recommends that music treatment can be a significant expansion to the treatment plan for individuals with a chemical imbalance, however, its viability might shift from one individual to another. It's fundamental to talk with a certified music specialist or medical services proficient for customized direction.

Correspondence Improvement: Music treatment can help people with chemical imbalances in putting themselves out there through non-verbal means. It energizes vocalizations, motions, and the utilization of instruments to convey.

Profound Guideline: Music can summon feelings and mindsets. Music treatment can assist people with chemical imbalances in dealing with their feelings, diminishing tension, and working on self-guideline abilities.

Interactive abilities: Gathering music treatment meetings can advance social connection and collaboration. Members figure out how to draw in with others through singing, playing instruments, and alternating.

Tangible Joining: Many individuals with mental imbalances have tactile awareness. Music treatment can assist with tangible joining bit by bit presenting people with various sounds and surfaces in a controlled and strong climate.

Individualized Approach: Music specialists tailor their intercessions to meet the particular requirements and inclinations of every person with a chemical imbalance. This customized approach augments the treatment's viability.

Evaluations and Objectives: Music advisors lead appraisals to distinguish qualities and regions that need improvement. They put forth clear objectives and track progress over the long haul.

Multidisciplinary Cooperation: Music specialists frequently team up with other medical services experts, instructors, and parental figures to guarantee a comprehensive way to deal with the singular's therapy plan.

Examination and Proof: While there is developing proof of the advantages of music treatment in mental imbalance, it means a lot to take note that results can shift. A few people might answer more decidedly than others.

Keep in mind, that music treatment is only one of many ways to deal with help people with mental imbalance. It ought to be coordinated into a far-reaching treatment plan that thinks about the singular's extraordinary requirements and inclinations. Talking with a certified music specialist or mental imbalance expert is essential for direction and suggestions custom-fitted to a particular case.

Art Therapy

Workmanship treatment can be advantageous for people with mental imbalances. It gives an imaginative outlet to self-articulation, correspondence, and close-to-home guidelines. Craftsmanship can assist people with chemical imbalances, foster fine-coordinated movements, work on friendly association, and lessen tension. It's crucial to work with a prepared craftsmanship specialist who can fit the meetings to the singular's necessities and inclinations.

Correspondence Help: For non-verbal or negligibly verbal people with mental imbalances, workmanship can act as an integral asset for correspondence. They can offer viewpoints, sentiments, and encounters through their fine art.

Tangible Combination: Workmanship treatment can address tactile awarenesses frequently found in mental imbalance. It permits people to investigate various surfaces, varieties, and materials, assisting with tangible reconciliation and guidelines.

Close to home Articulation: Numerous people with chemical imbalances battle with recognizing and communicating feelings. Making workmanship can help them investigate and impart their sentiments in a non-verbal manner.

Interactive abilities: Gathering workmanship treatment meetings can work on interactive abilities by empowering cooperation, sharing, and turn-taking among members. It gives an organized climate to rehearsing social communications.

Confidence: Finishing craftsmanship projects and getting positive criticism can support confidence and trust in people with mental imbalances.

Unwinding and Adapting: Workmanship can be an unwinding and quieting movement, assisting people with overseeing tension or tangible over burden.

Individualized Approach: Craftsmanship treatment ought to be customized to the singular's inclinations and necessities, taking into account their tangible responsive qualities and correspondence capacities.

Generally speaking, workmanship treatment can be an important expansion to the treatment plan for people with chemical imbalances, advancing self-articulation, close-to-home prosperity, and social turn of events.

Animal-Assisted Therapy

Workmanship treatment can be advantageous for people with mental imbalances. It gives an imaginative outlet to self-articulation, correspondence, and close-to-home guidelines. Craftsmanship can assist people with chemical imbalances, foster fine-coordinated movements, work on friendly association, and lessen tension. It's crucial to work with a prepared craftsmanship specialist who can fit the meetings to the singular's necessities and inclinations.

Correspondence Help: For non-verbal or negligibly verbal people with mental imbalances, workmanship can act as an integral asset for correspondence. They can offer viewpoints, sentiments, and encounters through their fine art.

Tangible Combination: Workmanship treatment can address tactile awarenesses frequently found in mental imbalance. It permits people to investigate various surfaces, varieties, and materials, assisting with tangible reconciliation and guidelines.

Close to home Articulation: Numerous people with chemical imbalances battle with recognizing and communicating feelings. Making workmanship can help them investigate and impart their sentiments in a non-verbal manner.

Interactive abilities: Gathering workmanship treatment meetings can work on interactive abilities by empowering cooperation, sharing, and turn-taking among members. It gives an organized climate to rehearsing social communications.

Confidence: Finishing craftsmanship projects and getting positive criticism can support confidence and trust in people with mental imbalances.

Unwinding and Adapting: Workmanship can be an unwinding and quieting movement, assisting people with overseeing tension or tangible over-burden.

Individualized Approach: Craftsmanship treatment ought to be customized to the singular's inclinations and necessities, taking into account their tangible responsive qualities and correspondence capacities.

Generally speaking, workmanship treatment can be an important expansion to the treatment plan for people with chemical imbalances, advancing self-articulation, close-to-home prosperity, and social turn of events.

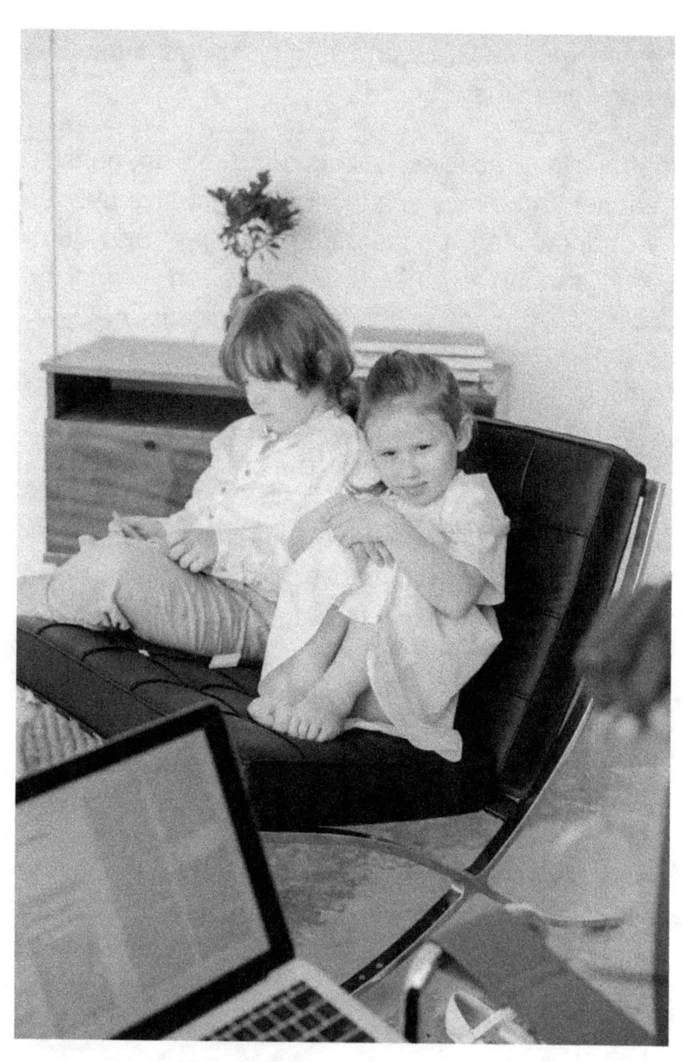

Chapter 8: Medical Interventions

Medications for Autism-Related Symptoms

There are no prescriptions that can fix the chemical imbalance, as it is a neurodevelopmental problem with a complicated and various scope of side effects. In any case, a few drugs might be recommended to assist with overseeing explicit mental imbalance-related side effects or co-happening conditions. These can include:

Antipsychotic Prescriptions: They might be recommended to oversee crabbiness, hostility, or self-harmful ways of behaving frequently connected with a chemical imbalance. Models incorporate risperidone and aripiprazole.

Particular Serotonin Reuptake Inhibitors (SSRIs): These antidepressants might be utilized to address tension and tedious ways of behaving in people with mental imbalance. Models incorporate fluoxetine and sertraline.

Energizers: Now and again, energizer prescriptions like methylphenidate or amphetamines might be endorsed to oversee hyperactivity or consideration issues that co-occur with chemical imbalance.

Against nervousness Drugs: Prescriptions like benzodiazepines or buspirone might be utilized to reduce tension side effects.

Melatonin: It's an enhancement, not a drug, but rather it tends to be utilized to assist direct rest designs in people with chemical imbalances who experience issues dozing.

Prescriptions for Comorbid Conditions: Here and there, people with chemical imbalances might have co-happening conditions like epilepsy or gastrointestinal issues. Meds well-defined for those conditions might be recommended.

It's vital to note that medicine choices ought to be made in consultation with medical services professionals who spend significant time in chemical imbalance, as every individual's necessities are special, and possible advantages and dangers ought to be painstakingly thought of. Moreover, conduct and restorative mediations are much of the time a significant piece of chemical imbalance treatment.

Dietary and Nutritional Considerations

Dietary and nourishing contemplations in chemical imbalance can assume a critical part in overseeing side effects and advancing in general prosperity. While individual requirements might change, here are a few central issues to consider:

Adjusted Diet: Guarantee the person with chemical imbalance consumes a decent eating routine wealthy in natural products, vegetables, lean proteins, and entire grains. A changed eating routine gives fundamental supplements.

Sans gluten and Without casein Diet (GF/CF): A few people with chemical imbalances might profit from a GF/CF diet, as they accept it can lessen specific side effects. In any case, logical proof supporting its viability is restricted, and it ought to be embraced under the direction of a medical services proficient.

Supplements: Examine with a medical services supplier whether enhancements like omega-3 unsaturated fats, vitamin D or probiotics are fundamental. These enhancements might uphold by and large well-being.

Food Responsive Qualities and Sensitivities: Know about any food awarenesses or sensitivities the individual might have. Kill trigger food varieties to forestall unfriendly responses.

Stomach-related Wellbeing: Address any stomach-related issues, as gastrointestinal issues are normal in certain people with chemical imbalances. Fiber-rich food varieties and probiotics can assist with keeping up with stomach wellbeing.

Surface and Tactile Inclinations: Consider tangible responsive qualities and food surfaces while arranging dinners. Offer food sources that line up with tangible inclinations to energize a more changed diet.

Routine and Design: Lay out a steady supper schedule, as people with chemical imbalances frequently blossom with consistency. This can diminish pressure connected with supper time.

Social Contemplations: A few dietary changes might influence conduct. Screen for any progressions and talk with experts on a case-by-case basis.

Meeting with a Dietitian: Look for direction from an enrolled dietitian or nutritionist experienced in working with people with mental imbalance. They can make customized dietary plans.

Hydration: Guarantee satisfactory hydration. Water is fundamental for general well-being and can assist with processing and by and large prosperity.

Recall that each person with mental imbalance is exceptional, and what works for one individual may not work for another. It's urgent to talk with medical care experts who can give customized directions in light of the singular's particular necessities and inclinations.

Alternative and Complementary Therapies

Option and integral treatments for chemical imbalance range jumble (ASD) are many times sought after by guardians and parental figures looking for extra help for their friends and family. It's vital to take note that the viability of these treatments changes, and not all have logical proof to help their utilization. Here are a few regularly investigated approaches:

Dietary Mediations: A few guardians attempt without gluten, sans casein (GFCF), or other specific weight control plans, accepting they might decrease mental imbalance side effects. Be that as it may, logical proof supporting these weight control plans is restricted, and they ought to be embraced with alertness.

Nutrients and Enhancements: Enhancements like vitamin B6, magnesium, and omega-3 unsaturated fats are some of the time utilized, yet research on their viability is uncertain. Talk with a medical care proficient before presenting supplements.

Social Treatments: Applied Conduct Investigation (ABA) is a broadly acknowledged social treatment for chemical imbalance. It centers around ability improvement and conducts the board.

Tangible-Based Treatments: Tactile joining treatment and word-related treatment can assist people with tangible responsive qualities or difficulties in managing tangible info.

Mind-Body Practices: A few families investigate rehearsals like yoga, contemplation, or needle therapy to assist with unwinding and stress the board, although their immediate effect on chemical imbalance side effects is muddled.

Hyperbaric Oxygen Treatment (HBOT): This includes taking in unadulterated oxygen in a compressed chamber. Research on HBOT's viability in treating chemical imbalances is restricted.

Elective Drugs: Homeopathy, natural cures, and other elective medicines are utilized by some, yet proof supporting their viability is for the most part inadequate.

It's vital to move toward these treatments with alertness and talk with medical care experts. What works for one person with mental imbalance may not work for another, and there is no one size-fits-all methodology. Proof-based mediation, for example, early intercession projects and language training, ought to stay focal in overseeing ASD. Continuously talk with a certified medical services supplier to settle on informed conclusions about other options and reciprocal treatments for chemical imbalances.

Sleep Management Strategies

Overseeing rest in people with mental imbalance can be challenging. Here are a few methodologies that might prove to be useful:

Reliable Everyday Practice: Lay out an ordinary rest plan with predictable sleep time and wake-up times to control the body's inner clock.

Establish an Agreeable Rest Climate: Guarantee the room hushes up, dim, and agreeable. Use power outage draperies, repetitive sounds, or quieting tactile things if necessary.

Limit Screen Time: Keep away from electronic gadgets before sleep time as the blue light can upset rest. Make a breeze down everyday practice with quieting exercises all things considered.

Tactile Contemplations: People with chemical imbalances might have tangible responsive qualities. Focus on sheet material materials, nightwear, and sleepwear to give solace.

Diet and Hydration: Stay away from weighty dinners, caffeine, and a lot of fluids near sleep time to forestall evening enlightenments.

Actual work: Empower ordinary active work during the day to advance better rest, however, stay away from overwhelming activity near sleep time.

Social Stories and Visual Timetables: Utilize visual guides and social stories to assist people with mental imbalances in comprehending and planning for sleep time schedules.

Unwinding Strategies: Show unwinding methods like profound breathing, moderate muscle unwinding, or care to decrease uneasiness and advance rest.

Melatonin: Counsel medical care proficient before considering melatonin supplements, as they might be fitting for certain people with mental imbalances.

Look for Proficient Assistance: If rest issues continue to happen, counsel a medical services supplier or expert who can resolve fundamental issues like rest problems or tactile responsive qualities.

Recall that every individual with mental imbalance is remarkable, so fitting the rest of the board procedures to their particular requirements and preferences is fundamental. Talking with medical care experts and social specialists can be useful in fostering a customized rest plan.

Chapter 9: Parental Care and Support

Parenting Strategies for Autism

Nurturing a youngster with chemical imbalance can be testing however fulfilling. Here are a few techniques:

Early Intercession: Look for early analysis and mediation administrations for your youngster.

Organized Everyday practice: Make an anticipated day-to-day schedule to assist your youngster with having a real sense of safety.

Clear Correspondence: Utilize visual guides, signals, and basic language to upgrade correspondence.

Uplifting feedback: The Prize wanted ways of behaving to support them.

Tangible Help: Figure out your youngster's tactile responsive qualities and give tangible well-disposed conditions.

Interactive abilities: Educate and rehearse interactive abilities through play and organized exercises.

Specific Schooling: Consider custom curriculum projects or treatments custom-made to chemical imbalance.

Support Gatherings: Associate with different guardians and care groups to share encounters and guidance.

Taking care of oneself: Deal with yourself to lessen pressure and be a superior guardian.

Persistence and Compassion: Show tolerance and sympathy to grasp your youngster's point of view.

Recall that each kid with mental imbalance is one of a kind, so tailor your way to deal with their particular requirements and qualities. Talking with experts can likewise give important direction.

Self-Care for Parents

Taking care of oneself is vital for guardians of kids with mental imbalances to oversee pressure and keep up with prosperity. Here are some ways to take care of oneself tips:

Look for Help: Associate with help gatherings, advisors, or different guardians of medically introverted youngsters for daily reassurance and counsel.

Plan "Personal" Time: Put away normal breaks to re-energize, regardless of whether it's only 15 minutes of calm time every day.

Keep an Everyday practice: Lay out a day-to-day timetable to make consistency for both you and your kid.

Sound Way of Life: Focus on rest, workout, and a decent eating regimen to keep up with physical and profound well-being.

Reprieve Care: Sort out for rest care to offer yourself a reprieve when required.

Care and Unwinding: Practice care procedures or reflection to decrease pressure.

Leisure activities and Interests: Set aside a few minutes for exercises you appreciate to support your advantages and interests.

Delegate and Request Help: Go ahead and family or companions for help when essential.

Teach Yourself: Consistently instruct yourself about mental imbalance to all the more likely comprehend and uphold your youngster.

Proficient Assistance: Consider treatment or guidance to assist you with adapting to the novel difficulties of nurturing a kid with a chemical imbalance.

Recollect that taking care of oneself isn't narrow-minded; it's fundamental for your prosperity and, at last, your capacity to give the best consideration to your youngster.

Sibling Support

Kin support in chemical imbalance is critical for cultivating grasping, compassion, and positive connections inside the family. Here are far to offer help:

Instruction: Assist kin with understanding what mental imbalance is, its attributes, and what it means for their medically introverted kin. Age-fitting assets and books can be helpful.

Correspondence: Empower transparent correspondence. Permit kin to clarify pressing issues and express their sentiments and concerns.

Quality Time: Invest one-on-one energy with every kin to reinforce their singular bonds and guarantee they don't feel dismissed.

Support Gatherings: Consider joining support gatherings or treatment meetings explicitly intended for kin of medically introverted people. It gives a place of refuge to share encounters.

Association: Remember kin for treatment meetings or chemical imbalance-related exercises when fitting. This inclusion can assist them with feeling more associated.

Tolerance and Figuring out: Show restraint toward kin's responses and feelings. Comprehend that they might encounter a scope of sentiments, including envy, disappointment, or pride.

Support Sympathy: Show compassion by examining how their mentally unbalanced kin might unexpectedly encounter the world. Urge them to be understanding and steady.

Individual Requirements: Perceive and address every kin's singular necessities and sentiments. No two kin will respond to the same approach to having a mentally unbalanced relative.

Rest Care: Sort out rest care or breaks for kin and guardians to lessen pressure and permit time for taking care of oneself.

Long haul Arranging: Examine likely arrangements, including providing care liabilities, with kin as they become older to guarantee everybody is in total agreement.

Kin backing can essentially influence the prosperity of both the mentally unbalanced individual and their kin, advancing an agreeable family climate.

Coordinating Care with Healthcare Professionals

Planning care for people with mental imbalance includes joint effort among different medical services experts and trained professionals. Here are a few vital stages and contemplations:

Essential Consideration Doctor: Begin with an essential consideration doctor who can give general medical care and references to trained professionals. They can supervise the general soundness of the person with mental imbalance.

Mental imbalance Subject matter experts: Search out mental imbalance trained professionals, like formative pediatricians, youngster specialists, or pediatric nervous system specialists, who can analyze and give direction on unambiguous mediations.

Conduct Advisors: Applied Conduct Investigation (ABA) specialists and other social specialists can give fitted mediations to address conduct difficulties.

Discourse and Language Advisors: Discourse language pathologists can assist with correspondence hardships frequently found in people with mental imbalances.

Word-related Advisors: Word-related specialists can address tangible responsive qualities and assist with growing fine and gross coordinated abilities.

Clinicians/Therapists: Emotional well-being experts can offer help for co-happening psychological well-being conditions that people with mental imbalance might insight into, like tension or wretchedness.

Custom curriculum Experts: If the individual is young, team up with specialized curriculum educators, language teachers, and different teachers to make an Individualized Training Plan (IEP).

ABA Bosses: Assuming ABA treatment is essential for the treatment plan, coordinate with the ABA manager to guarantee consistency and progress.

Care Coordination Group: Consider a consideration facilitator or caseworker who can assist with sorting out arrangements, speak with various experts, and guarantee a comprehensive way to deal with care.

Family and Parental figure Contribution: Keep relatives and guardians engaged with the consideration plan, as they assume an urgent part in the singular's day-to-day routine and progress.

Standard Correspondence: Guarantee that all experts associated with the singular's consideration impart consistently to share updates, objectives, and acclimations to the treatment plan.

Change Arranging: As the person with mental imbalance develops, plan for advances, for example, from pediatric to grown-up care or from school to post-school administrations.

Advocate for the Person: Be a backer for the person with a mental imbalance, guaranteeing their necessities are met and their privileges are regarded inside the medical care framework.

Remain Informed: Stay up with the latest with the most recent explorations and treatments connected with a chemical imbalance to settle on informed conclusions about treatment choices.

Recall that every person with a chemical imbalance is novel, and their consideration plan ought to be custom-made to their particular necessities and qualities. Powerful coordination among medical services experts is fundamental to giving thorough and all-encompassing consideration.

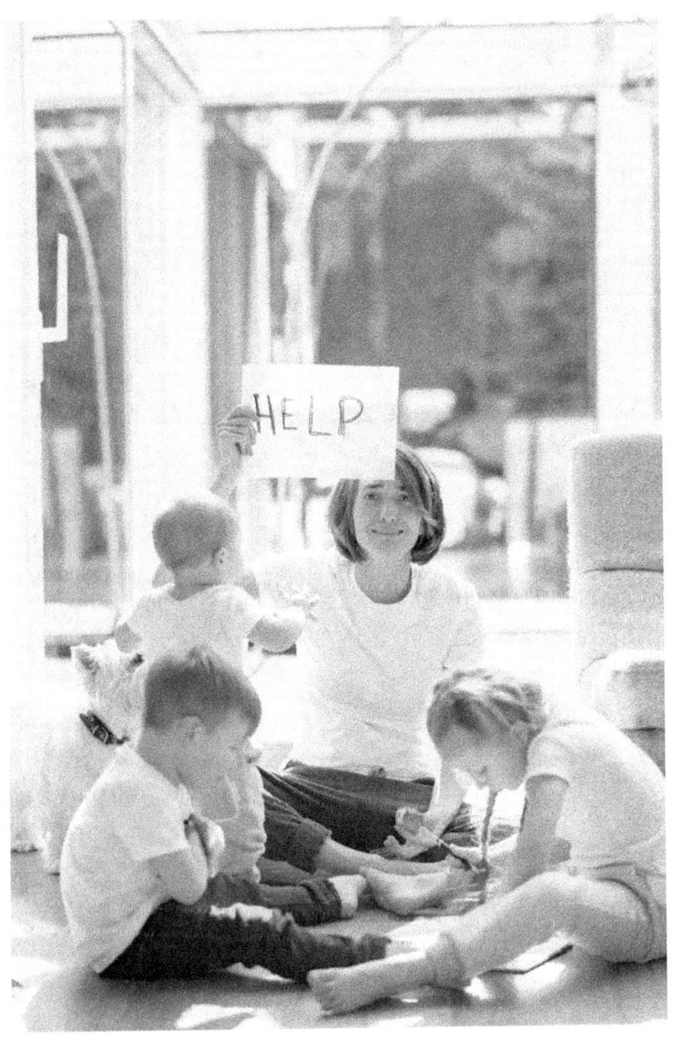
HELP

Chapter 10: Advocacy and Resources

Empowering Parents as Advocates

Enabling guardians as backers in mental imbalance is vital for guaranteeing that people with chemical imbalances get the help and assets they need. This can include:

Schooling: Giving guardians data about mental imbalance range jumble (ASD) so they can all the more likely figure out their kid's necessities and freedoms.

Support Gatherings: Making encouraging groups of people were guardians can share encounters, systems, and guidance.

Backing Preparing: Furnishing guardians with the ability to explore the instructive and medical care frameworks to get fitting administrations for their kids.

Strategy Support: Empowering guardians to take part in backing at neighborhood, state, and public levels to advance arrangements that benefit people with chemical imbalances.

Local area Contribution: Empowering guardians to take part in mental imbalance-related occasions and exercises to bring issues to light and decrease shame.

Enabling guardians can prompt superior results and a more comprehensive society for people with mental imbalances.

Connecting with Support Groups

To associate with help bunches for a chemical imbalance, you can attempt the accompanying advances:

Online Assets: Quest for mental imbalance support bunches on sites, discussions, and virtual entertainment stages like Facebook or Reddit. Many gatherings offer a place of refuge for people and families impacted by a mental imbalance to interface and offer encounters.

Nearby Mental imbalance Associations: Contact neighborhood chemical imbalance associations or sections of public associations like Mental Imbalance Talks or the Chemical Imbalance Society. They frequently have support gatherings and can give data on gatherings and occasions in your space.

Mental imbalance Centers and Advisors: Contact chemical imbalance facilities, advisors, and experts in your district. They might have the option to suggest neighborhood support gatherings or deal assets for associating with others locally.

Schools and Instructive Foundations: If you have a kid with a mental imbalance, your kid's school or instructive establishment might have data about nearby care groups or parent organizations.

Online Care Groups: Consider joining the web support gatherings and networks committed to chemical imbalance. These can give significant data, counsel, and a feeling of having a place. Sites like Mental Imbalance Talks and Wrong Planet deal with such assets.

Go to Mental imbalance-related Occasions: Go to gatherings, studios, and classes connected with chemical imbalance in your space. These occasions frequently give chances to arrange other people who share comparable encounters.

Ask Medical Services Experts: Talk with your kid's pediatrician or mental imbalance experts for proposals on neighborhood support gatherings or assets.

Recall that the accessibility of care groups might differ depending on your area, so be constant in your hunt and connect with various hotspots for help.

Accessing Government and Community Resources

Getting to government and local area assets for mental imbalance can fluctuate by area, however, here are some general moves toward the beginning:

Contact Nearby Government Offices: Connect with your neighborhood government's wellbeing or social administration division. They can give data on accessible projects, administrations, and financing choices.

School Locale Administrations: If you have a kid with a chemical imbalance, contact your school region's custom curriculum division. They can assist with instructive help and assessments.

Health care coverage: Audit your health care coverage strategy to comprehend what chemical imbalance-related administrations are covered. Numerous approaches cover treatments like ABA (Applied Conduct Investigation).

Mental imbalance Support Gatherings: Associate with mental imbalance backing associations in your space. They frequently have assets, support gatherings, and data on neighborhood administrations.

Online Assets: Investigate sites like Chemical Imbalance Talks, the Mental Imbalance Society, and the Chemical Imbalance Self-Backing Organization for data, assets, and backing.

Early Mediation Projects: If you have a small kid with a chemical imbalance, ask about early mediation programs in your space. These can be basic for an early turn of events.

Advisors and Trained professionals: Look for suggestions from advisors, discourse pathologists, word-related specialists, and different experts who work with people with chemical imbalances.

Support Gatherings: Join nearby mental imbalance support gatherings or online networks. These can give significant data and basic encouragement.

Monetary Help: Ask about monetary help programs for people with disabilities, like Supplemental Security Pay (SSI) or Medicaid.

Lawful and Promotion Backing: If necessary, talk with legitimate experts who spend significant time in handicap privileges and support.

Recall that the accessibility of assets can shift extraordinarily by locale, so exploring what's particularly accessible in your area is significant. Furthermore, consider making a customized plan given your or your cherished one's remarkable necessities.

Legal Rights and Disability Services

Legitimate privileges and inability administrations for people with chemical imbalance can differ by nation and locale, however, a few normal standards and assets exist:

Hostile to Segregation Regulations: Numerous nations have regulations that restrict the victimization of people with incapacities, including chemical imbalance. For instance, in the US, the Americans with Handicaps Act (ADA) gives legitimate assurances.

Schooling Privileges: In many spots, youngsters with chemical imbalances reserve the option to get proper training in all prohibitive climates. This might include administrations like custom curriculum, language instruction, or word-related treatment.

Individualized Training Plan (IEP): In the U.S., an IEP is a legitimately restricting report that frames the instructive administrations and facilities an understudy with mental imbalance ought to get in school.

Admittance to Medical Care: Admittance to medical care administrations and treatments is critical for people with chemical imbalances. A nation has explicit projects or protection arrangements to assist with taking care of these expenses.

Social Administrations: Different social administrations can help people with mental imbalance and their families, including professional preparation, lodging backing, and relief care.

Backing Gatherings: Mental imbalance promotion associations can give data and backing on legitimate privileges and accessible administrations. Models incorporate the Mental Imbalance Society of America and Chemical Imbalance Talks.

Legitimate Guardianship: In situations where people with mental imbalance will be unable to settle on specific choices autonomously, lawful guardianship or conservatorship might be important to safeguard their privileges and prosperity.

Work Privileges: Numerous nations have regulations that safeguard people with handicaps from business separation. Sensible facilities might be expected in the working environment.

Assistive Innovation: Lawful freedoms may likewise incorporate admittance to assistive advancements that can assist people with mental imbalance and work all the more autonomously.

It's vital to research and figure out the particular regulations and administrations accessible in your locale, as they can change altogether. Talking with neighborhood handicap promotion associations or lawful specialists who spend significant time on inability privileges can be useful for exploring these intricacies.

Chapter 11: Social Skills and Relationships

Building Friendships and Social Connections

Building companionships and social associations for people with chemical imbalances can be fulfilling however in some cases the testing process is. Here are a few hints to help:

Figure out Chemical imbalance: Teach yourself as well as other people about mental imbalance to expand mindfulness and comprehension of the condition.

Join Care Groups: Search out nearby or online mental imbalance support bunches where you can associate with other people who share comparable encounters.

Foster Interactive abilities: Energize interactive ability advancement through treatment or interactive abilities bunches custom-fitted to people with a chemical imbalance.

Distinguish Interests: Find exercises or leisure activities that line up with the singular's advantages, as shared interests can be an establishment for kinships.

Work on Mingling: Practice social communications through pretending or organized situations to assemble certainty.

Utilize Visual Backings: Visual backings like social stories or timetables can assist people with chemical imbalances in exploring social circumstances.

Show restraint: Comprehend that building connections might require some investment and require persistence. Be available for continuous advancement.

Energize Correspondence: Backing compelling correspondence, which can be verbal or non-verbal, contingent upon the singular's capacities.

Set Sensible Assumptions: Perceive that not all people with chemical imbalance will have similar social objectives or capacities, so set reasonable assumptions.

Advanced Inclusivity: Empower comprehensive conditions where contrasts are embraced, and everybody feels acknowledged.

Peer Coaching: Consider peer tutoring programs where neurotypical people can get to know and support those with chemical imbalances.

Take part in Exceptional Interests: Take part in exercises and gatherings connected with the singular's extraordinary advantages, which can open doors to association.

Advance Freedom: Support independence and navigation, enabling people with chemical imbalances to step up to the plate in friendly circumstances.

Expect Tactile Requirements: Be aware of tangible responsive qualities and establish conditions that oblige them.

Look for Proficient Assistance: If difficulties continue, talk with experts, for example, analysts or advisors, who have some expertise in mental imbalance.

Recall that building companionships and social associations is a one-of-a-kind excursion for every person with mental imbalance. Tailor your way to deal with their particular necessities and inclinations while cultivating a strong and grasping local area.

Addressing Bullying and Teasing

Addressing bullying and teasing of individuals with autism is crucial. Here are some steps to help:

Education: Raise awareness about autism to promote understanding and empathy among peers.

Communication: Encourage open dialogue with the person with autism to understand their feelings and experiences.

Reporting: Encourage bystanders to report bullying incidents to teachers or authorities.

School Policies: Ensure schools have strong anti-bullying policies in place and enforce them consistently.

Support: Offer emotional support and counseling to both the person with autism and the bullies.

Social Skills: Provide social skills training to help individuals with autism navigate social situations better.

Inclusion: Promote inclusive activities and friendships to reduce isolation.

Parent Involvement: Engage parents in addressing bullying and teasing issues with the school.

Peer Training: Conduct peer education programs to teach students about autism and foster acceptance.

Role Modeling: Encourage positive role modeling among peers and adults.

Combating bullying requires a community effort to create a safe and inclusive environment for everyone.

Developing Age-Appropriate Relationships

Creating age-fitting connections in people with chemical imbalances can be a nuanced cycle that requires grasping, support, and customized methodologies. Here are a few key contemplations:

Interactive abilities Preparing: Numerous people with chemical imbalances benefit from organized interactive abilities preparing programs. These projects can show significant abilities, for example, starting discussions, perusing meaningful gestures, and figuring out non verbal correspondence.

Peer-Interceded Intercessions: Empowering connections with neurotypical friends can be significant. Peer-interceded intercessions include educating neurotypical peers about mental imbalance and encouraging comprehensive social conditions.

Individualized Approach: Perceive that every individual with a chemical imbalance is novel, with their assets and difficulties. Tailor systems to their particular requirements and inclinations.

Correspondence Backing: For those with restricted verbal correspondence, augmentative and elective correspondence (AAC) frameworks can work with social cooperation.

Tangible Contemplations: Numerous people with mental imbalances have tactile-responsive qualities. It's fundamental to establish tangible cordial conditions and think about tactile inclinations in friendly exercises.

Social Stories: Social stories and visual backings can assist people with chemical imbalances in grasping social assumptions and exploring different social circumstances.

Expanding on Interests: Gain by the singular's exceptional advantages as a method for interfacing with peers who share comparable interests.

Job Displaying: Positive good examples can be compelling in exhibiting suitable social ways of behaving. These can be companions, kin, or tutors.

Tolerance and Understanding: Persistence is vital while supporting people with mental imbalances in building connections. Celebrate little triumphs and comprehend mishaps.

Progress Arranging: As people with chemical imbalances change into pre-adulthood and adulthood, it means a lot to make arrangements for their developing social necessities and likely heartfelt connections.

Family Contribution: Families assume a fundamental part in supporting the social turn of events. Team up with families to build up abilities mastered in treatment at home.

Proficient Direction: Look for direction from experts experienced in working with a mental imbalance, like language teachers, word-related advisors, and conduct specialists.

Recall that building age-fitting connections is a steady cycle, and advance might fluctuate for every person. Stressing consideration, sympathy, and understanding can go quite far in supporting people with chemical imbalances in their social turn of events.

Chapter 12: Sensory Integration

Sensory Diet and Sensory Activities

A tactile eating routine is a customized plan of tangible exercises and procedures intended to help people, incorporating those with chemical imbalances, control their tangible encounters. Tactile exercises can be valuable for people with mental imbalance by giving tangible information that helps them self-direct and oversee tangible responsive qualities. Here are a few normal tangible exercises utilized in tactile weight control plans for people with chemical imbalances:

Profound Tension: Exercises like weighted covers, profound strain back rubs, or pressure pieces of clothing can give quieting profound touch pressure.

Proprioceptive Exercises: These exercises include developments and activities that draw in the muscles and joints, like hopping on a trampoline, hard work, or pushing/pulling objects.

Vestibular Exercises: Swinging, turning, or shaking can invigorate the vestibular framework and help with a tactile combination.

Material Exercises: Exercises that include different surfaces, for example, playing with tangible receptacles loaded up with rice or sand, finger painting, or utilizing finished toys, can be valuable.

Visual Exercises: Visual excitement can shift from watching quiet recordings or utilizing tactile lighting to decrease tangible over-burden.

Hearable Exercises: Controlled openness to hearable upgrades, such as standing by listening to quieting music or background noise, assist people with directing their hear-able awarenesses.

Oral Tactile Exercises: Biting gum, utilizing bite toys, or sucking on hard confections can give oral tangible info.

It's essential to work with a word-related advisor or tactile expert to make a tangible eating routine custom-fitted to a singular's particular necessities and responsive qualities. The objective is to assist the singular in better adapting to tangible difficulties and further develop their general prosperity and working.

Sensory Integration Therapy

Tangible Reconciliation Treatment (SIT) is a methodology frequently utilized for people with chemical imbalance range jumble (ASD) to assist them with better handling tactile data. It includes exercises that open people to different tangible upgrades to work on their tactile handling and guidelines. While certain people with ASD might profit from SIT, its viability fluctuates from one individual to another. It's fundamental to talk with a certified specialist or medical care proficient who can evaluate and fit the treatment to meet the particular requirements of the person with a chemical imbalance. Remember that there are other proof-based medications and treatments accessible for people with chemical imbalances, so a customized approach is essential.

Objectives of SIT: The essential objective of SIT is to assist people with mental imbalance and answer tangible data in a more versatile manner. It intends to address tactile difficulties regularly experienced by people with ASD, like excessive touchiness (going overboard to tangible information) or hyposensitivity (underreacting to tangible information).

Tactile Info: SIT includes presenting people with different tangible data sources, including contact, sound, development, and visual improvements, in an organized and restorative way. These tactile exercises are intended to assist people with turning out to be more agreeable and less receptive to tangible encounters.

Helpful Exercises: SIT meetings might incorporate exercises like swinging, brushing, profound strain kneading, skipping on a treatment ball, or drawing in with finished materials. These exercises are custom-fitted to the person's tangible profile and needs.

Qualified Specialists: SIT ought to be led via prepared word-related advisors or different experts with ability in the tactile mix. They survey the person's tangible handling of challenges and make a customized treatment plan.

Examination and Viability: While some episodic proof proposes benefits, the logical proof supporting SIT for chemical imbalance is blended. A few investigations have shown positive results, while others have not. It's fundamental to consider other proof-based mediations like Applied Conduct

Investigation (ABA), language instruction, and interactive abilities are prepared close by SIT.

Individualized Approach: Chemical imbalance is a range problem, and every individual's tangible difficulties are extraordinary. Consequently, the viability of SIT can shift broadly. It's significant to screen progress and change the treatment on a case-by-case basis.

Parent Contribution: Guardians and guardians frequently assume a critical part in supporting tangible combination exercises at home. They can work with advisors to learn systems for advancing tangible guidelines.

Elective Treatments: notwithstanding SIT, a few people with mental imbalance benefit from different treatments like music treatment, craftsmanship treatment, or creature-helped treatment, which can likewise address tangible necessities.

In synopsis, Tactile Combination Treatment can be a significant device in assisting people with chemical imbalances to oversee tangible difficulties, yet it's vital to approach it as a component of a thorough treatment plan customized to the singular's one-of-a-kind necessities and inclinations. Meeting with medical services experts and specialists experienced in mental imbalance is vital to deciding the most appropriate medications.

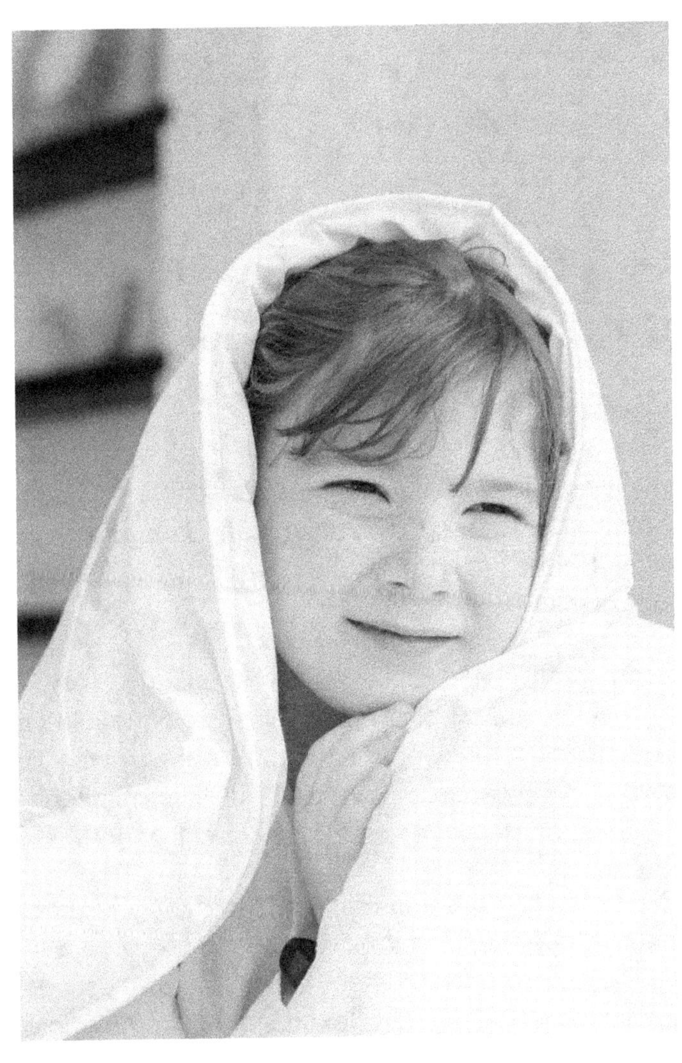

Chapter: 13 Assistive Technology

Using Technology for Communication and Learning

Involving innovation for correspondence and learning in mental imbalance can be profoundly helpful. Here are a few different ways innovation can help:

Augmentative and Elective Correspondence (AAC) Applications: AAC applications like Proloquo2Go or TouchChat empower non-verbal people with a mental imbalance to impart utilizing images, pictures, or messages on a tablet or cell phone.

Discourse-to-Text and Text-to-Discourse Devices: These apparatuses can help people who battle with verbal correspondence. Discourse-to-message applications decipher expressed words into messages, while message-to-discourse applications convert messages into discourse.

Visual Timetables and Social Stories: Applications can assist with making visual timetables and social stories, which are fundamental for people with mental imbalances to grasp schedules and social circumstances.

Instructive Applications: Numerous instructive applications take special care of different learning styles and can assist people with chemical imbalances foster scholarly abilities and grow their insight in a tomfoolery and connecting way.

Virtual Learning Conditions: These stages work with web-based getting the hang of, permitting people with mental imbalance to get to schooling and treatment benefits from a distance.

Wearable Gadgets: A few wearable gadgets are intended to screen and oversee tangible responsive qualities and profound states, giving important bits of knowledge to parental figures and specialists.

Teletherapy: Teletherapy stages offer remote admittance to discourse, word-related, and social treatment, making it more helpful for people with a chemical imbalance and their families.

Interactive abilities Applications: Applications like "Social Express" or "Model Me Children" give intuitive examples and reproductions to show interactive abilities and profound guidelines.

Tactile Applications: These applications can assist people with tangible responsive qualities by giving quieting visuals and sounds, and supporting self-guideline.

Online Help People group: Innovation empowers people with a chemical imbalance and their families to interface with others confronting comparative difficulties, encouraging a feeling of the local area and sharing important data.

It's fundamental to survey every individual's novel requirements and inclinations to figure out which innovation instruments and applications are generally appropriate for their correspondence and learning objectives. Furthermore, proficient direction from specialists and teachers can be important in choosing and executing these advances.

Apps and Devices for Autism

There are different applications and gadgets intended to help people with chemical imbalances. Here are a few models:

Applications:

Proloquo2Go: A correspondence application with images and text-to-discourse for non-verbal people.

Mental imbalance Tracker Genius: Helps track and oversee ways of behaving, feelings, and schedules.

Visual Timetable Organizer: Makes visual timetables to assist with day-to-day schedules.

Tangible Applications: Applications like "Inhale, Think, Do with Sesame" can support close-to-home guidelines.

Social Stories Maker and Library: Creates social stories to show interactive abilities.

Gadgets:

AAC Gadgets: Augmentative and Elective Specialized gadgets like Tobii Dynavox give discourse support.

Tactile Devices: Instruments like twirly gigs or weighted covers can assist with tangible necessities.

Surrounding sound blocking Earphones: Valuable for people delicate to sound.

Tablets and PCs: Stacked with instructive applications and specialized devices.

Wearable Gadgets: Some smartwatches have applications for following feelings and ways of behaving.

Recollect that the adequacy of these devices can shift from one individual to another, so tweaking answers for a singular's necessities and preferences is fundamental. Continuously talk with a medical care or instructive expert for customized proposals.

Chapter 14: Transition to Adulthood

Preparing for Adolescence and Adulthood

Getting ready for pre-adulthood and adulthood for people with mental imbalance includes a blend of methodologies and backing to assist them with exploring the difficulties and open doors that accompany growing up. Here are a few key contemplations:

Early Intercession: Early mediation administrations are pivotal for kids with chemical imbalances. These administrations can incorporate language instruction, and word-related treatment, and conduct treatment to address explicit difficulties and fabricate fundamental abilities.

Individualized Instruction Plan (IEP): Team up with your kid's school to foster an IEP custom-fitted to their novel necessities. This plan can give facilities, custom curriculum administrations, and objectives that help their development.

Interactive abilities Preparing: Youths with chemical imbalances might profit from interactive abilities preparing to work on their capacity to collaborate with peers, make companions, and explore social circumstances.

Change Arranging: As your youngster approaches adulthood, start progress arranging early. This might include investigating professional and instructive open doors, autonomous living abilities, and occupation preparation programs.

Restorative Help: Proceed with treatment and backing administrations on a case-by-case basis, even into adulthood. Social treatment and different mediations can be significant all through an individual's life.

Self-Support: Show your youngster self-promotion abilities so they can communicate their necessities, inclinations, and objectives successfully.

Local area Commitment: Energize contribution in local area exercises and gatherings that line up with your kid's advantages and capacities.

Family Backing: Guarantee that your family approaches assets and encourages groups of people, for example, mental imbalance support gatherings and guiding administrations.

Clinical Consideration: Proceed with ordinary clinical check-ups and talk with medical services suppliers who have practical experience in chemical imbalance-related care.

Lawful and Monetary Preparation: Think about legitimate and monetary making arrangements for the future, for example, guardianship and exceptional necessities trusts.

Recall that each person with a chemical imbalance is special, and their requirements and assets might change. Tailor your way to deal with their particular circumstance, and look for direction from experts with skill in mental imbalance range problems as you explore the change to immaturity and adulthood.

Vocational Training and Employment

Professional preparation and work are valuable open doors for people with mental imbalance to stand out as of late. Here are a few central issues to consider:

Custom-made Projects: Professional preparation projects ought to be tweaked to meet the exceptional necessities and qualities of people with mental imbalances. This could include creating specific educational plans and instructing strategies.

Expertise Advancement: Spotlight on creating both occupation-explicit abilities and fundamental abilities, like correspondence, using time effectively, and interactive abilities, to upgrade employability.

Work Coordinating: Securing the right position match is critical. Distinguishing jobs that line up with a singular's advantages and assets can prompt more prominent work fulfillment and achievement.

Strong Workplace: Establishing a comprehensive and steady workplace is fundamental. Managers and collaborators ought to be taught about mental imbalance to encourage understanding and acknowledgment.

Work Training: Numerous people with chemical imbalances benefit from continuous work instructing and backing to assist them with exploring the work environment and addressing difficulties.

Remote Work Potential Open doors: Remote work can be a suitable choice for certain people with a mental imbalance, as it can give a more agreeable and controlled workplace.

Support and Mindfulness: Backing gatherings and mindfulness crusades assume a huge part in advancing equivalent work potential to open doors for people with mental imbalance.

Government Drives: Numerous nations have acquainted strategies and motivating forces to empower the employment of people with inabilities, including mental imbalance.

Progress Arranging: Change administrations in training ought to incorporate professionals wanting to guarantee a smooth change from school to business.

Learned: Energize deep-rooted acquiring and ability advancement to adjust to changing position markets and profession valuable open doors.

It's critical to perceive that every person with mental imbalance is one of a kind, so a customized way to deal with professional preparation and work is fundamental for progress.

Independent Living Skills

Autonomous living abilities are fundamental for people with mental imbalances to advance their independence and personal satisfaction. These abilities can include:

Relational abilities: Creating successful correspondence, both verbal and non-verbal, is significant for communicating needs and inclinations.

Taking care of oneself: Learning individual cleanliness schedules, dressing autonomously, and overseeing fundamental taking care of oneself undertakings.

Cooking and Nourishment: Showing dinner readiness, pursuing quality food decisions, and grasping dietary requirements.

Family Tasks: Empower cooperation in family errands like cleaning, clothing, and association.

Cash The board: Educating planning, saving, and fundamental monetary abilities.

Transportation: Showing how to utilize public transportation or drive a vehicle if pertinent.

Using time productively: Figuring out how to oversee timetables, arrangements, and obligations.

Interactive abilities: Creating social collaboration abilities, like making companions, grasping feelings, and perceiving meaningful gestures.

Critical thinking: Improving critical abilities to think to deal with regular difficulties.

Self-support: Training people to communicate their requirements and freedoms.

It's critical to offer individualized help and consider the particular requirements and capacities of every individual with chemical imbalance while chipping away at these abilities. Experts, parental figures, and advisors can assume critical parts in working on the improvement of these abilities.